MW01253694

ACTS OF THE BODY

TRILOGY ON PATHOLOGIES OF NARCISSISM RELATED TO THE BODY

PSYCHOLOGY OF EMOTIONS, MOTIVATIONS AND ACTIONS

Additional books in this series can be found on Nova's website under the Series tab.

Additional e-books in this series can be found on Nova's website under the e-book tab.

PSYCHOLOGY OF EMOTIONS, MOTIVATIONS AND ACTIONS

ACTS OF THE BODY

TRILOGY ON PATHOLOGIES OF NARCISSISM RELATED TO THE BODY

LÉLA CHIKHANI-NACOUZ
HÉLÈNE ISSA
AND
MOUNIR CHALHOUB

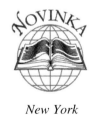

New York

NOTICE TO THE READER

Library of Congress Cataloging-in-Publication Data
The acts of the body : trilogy on pathologies of narcissism related to the body / authors, Lila Chikhani-Nacouz (Lebanese University II (Fanar), Psychotherapist, Beirut, Lebanon), Hilhne Issa (Balamand University, Beirut, Lebanon) and Mounir Chalhoub (BEING LCTC, Centre for Psychotherapy, Beirut, Lebanon).
    pages cm
 Includes index.
 ISBN 978-1-62417-622-7 (soft cover)
 1. Narcissism. I. Chikhani-Nacouz, Lila.
 BF575.N35A28 2013
 158.2--dc23
                    2013007530

Published by Nova Science Publishers, Inc. † New York

CONTENTS

FOREWORD

The profane body is currently collectivized and submitted to social principles of modeling of both behaviors and appearances. The body thus belongs to the public space. It is the subject and object of fundamental laws (needs to fill, freedom to grant, intimacy to preserve, jouissance to accord, health to safeguard, etc.), and the object and the subject of economic and commercial projects (modeling, publicity, fashion, sports games, etc.).

In this social space of appearance, strategies are elaborated around the representativeness of the body that multiply and compete. The image that we offer has first been the conception of a team, strategist, doctor, chemist, esthetician, visagiste, designer, fashion designer, journalist, businessman, and many others. The corporeal personality is of a young person, healthy, well cut, high stature, neat and hygienic. Constructing the body, the new elixir of youth, is a constant struggle for the appropriation of the self against aging and death, and the appropriation of the other's gaze. This narcissistic over-investment is the meaning granted to the modern conception of the corporeal fact. Commercialization and the management of corporeal appearances is a sociological inscription that modifies the meaning of the Ego and the world.

The modern world has loaded the body with a heavy burden. On the one hand, society individualizes it, but on the other it reshapes and rebuilds it in a homogenization of anatomies. Wanting to free his body of past traditions, modern man alienates it with modern traditions. *New pathologies* are related to the acts exerted on the body. They include the subject of this book: *bodybuildism*, *tattooism*, and *mummifism*, each of which qualifies as corporeal narcissism.

PREFACE

This work addresses the trilogy of the body: *Bodybuildism* (practicing sport to excess with an associated dependence on anabolic steroids and the consumption of hyper protein supplements), *tattooism* (a neologism to signify the behavior of marking the skin to excess, with more than one-third of the body surface tattooed), and *mummifism* (excessive packing of the infant for more than a year), as narcissistic pathology of the relational dynamics of the ego and body and/or of the skin.

These inscriptions are thought of as an identificatory corporealized language, and a substitute for parental disavowal. It is the study of the anaclitic processes of (I) the *bodybuilder* body image, (II) the space-skin *tattooist*, in the narcissistic identificatory processes, and the strategies put in place during the passage to the act; and (III) the virtuality of the image of the ego in the mummified skin and rigidified body, of the *mummifized* adolescent, in order to clarify, in these passages to the act, the formation of a doubled imago of the adolescent's body.

In order to implement this work, we adopted a similar method in the three processes studied.

- Semi-structured clinical interviews with 18 bodybuilders ranging between the ages of 15 and 20 (16 boys and 2 girls) and the administration of TAT to a male bodybuilder (18 years old) and a female bodybuilder (17 years old).
- Semi-structured clinical interviews with 11 *tattooists* ranging in age from 15to 20 (8 girls and 3 boys) and the administration of TAT to a female tattooist (19 years old) and a male tattooist (18 years old);

–   Semi-structured clinical interviews with six *mummifists* ranging between the ages of 15 and 20 (4 girls and 2 boys) and the administration of TAT to a mummifized girl (16 years old), and a mummifized boy (15 years old).

Due to the relatively small sample sizes, it is not possible to generalize the results. However, there are certain observations that can be made about these adolescents.

a)   There is a failure in the structuring of the body image. The adolescent attaches himself to the image of narcissistic misrecognition: the Ego is the image and not the image, the image of me.
b)   An unsatisfactory object relationship (splitter mother and defective father), implying an incompleteness in the subjectivation.
c)   A narcissistic and corporealized ideal ego leading to disorders on the imaginary register.
d)   A doubling of the imagos of the body: the archaic image and the acquired image by the passage to the act.

The excessive act of the body leads to a form of depersonalization of the adolescent with a corporealized ego, and refers him to a borderline narcissistic state.

INTRODUCTION

"Material of identity on the individual and collective level, the body is the space that is to be seen and read at the appreciation of others. It is through it that we are named, recognized, and identified as belonging to a social entity" [1: 13].

The body expresses and is expressed. Once there is insufficiency in the linguistic and gestural referential, the rest of the body takes precedence. It somatizes, it gets bigger, it weakens, it transforms, and it undergoes surgery. It can also be muscled or decorated.

This body, worked, refined, bared, muscled, tattooed and aestheticized is the expression of being, of the cultural and the symbolic. In the society of fashion, being exposed is an infatuation. It is for everyone to make a theater of his body. This *mise en scène* of the corporeality is a component of self-representations. The body is the site and the privileged expression of the relation of the Ego to ego and of Ego to the other.

The body changes of puberty, whether early or late, are a mandatory passage, which does violence to the body and the psyche of the adolescent. Access to genitality is often experienced as a violent attack. The body becomes a foreign body representing the objectal world, revealing flaws of childhood, and no longer protects the ego's boundaries and its intimacy. The anguish of castration leads youth to divert identificatory processes from their aim. What characterizes the adolescent is the back and forth movement between the investment of the object and narcissistic centration. This struggle, the result of unresolved previous conflicts, is combined with the fragility of object relations and identificatory benchmarks that constitute the subject's identity. To defend against the threat of intrusion of the Ego, the adolescent in distress, seeking self-image and identity, can foresee a solution through acting out the conflict. If the adolescent in crisis can drive himself towards delinquency, he can also be directed to processes of acting that are more addictive.

The passage to the act, in effect, seems to be a privileged means for the adolescent because it is favored by the narcissistic chasm, the instinctual emergence, the weakening of repression, and the vulnerability of the worsened Ego. These weaknesses do not allow - or allow only with difficultly - the implementation of secondary processes of defense. The regression to act becomes a type of safeguard. In fact, the involvement of adolescents in a practice can therefore be read as an open road to the exercise of the tendency that consists of the expulsion out of the psyche of affective contents or representatives that are sensed as persecutors or traumatic.

The addiction to act upon the body reflects the necessity of the body to appear. In this context, an excessive practice can be the palliative for the failure of the Ego functions. The Ego regresses to invest sensor motor and perceptual systems in a para-excitatory attempt to fight against the anguish produced. Physical sensations replace mental representations and absent affects. The passage to the act upon the corporeal would thus has the value of protecting the identity of the subject who practices it by marking the limits that he immediately imposes onto the body with which an object relation is tied, but in fact it just develops a corporeal narcissism.

Intensive training, endlessly repeated, for example, will lead the *bodybuilder* to forge an ideal body. This ideal body is consistent with the requirements of his practice, under the primacy of perceptible beauty. The repetition of notches on the skin leads the *tattooist* to forge a brand's name, an identity of substitution and a familial and social recognition. The body becomes a true body-machine or body-canvas, destined for exposure to the gazes: a corporeal sculpture or a painting is born in tribute to the affected narcissism.

When the display and marking become excessive, outrageous, repetitive, and their reason for being, they express a regressive return to the past, an identity mark that is imprinted on the skin and body. It is not discursive, but ritualized and sacred, acquired by the self, through arduous effort due to the failure to have a given identity. That stigma is indeed language, but a language of substitution for the failure of self-recognition.

The body and skin of substitution are second organs of replacement for the lack of the other, and the function of containing, both internally and externally, and are intended to substitute for the dependence on the primary object with a pseudo self-dependence through identificatory processes. The subject invests the setting up of a new body or a new skin on whose presence he will feel the need to check through repetition in order to feel his own existence in the will of restoring his narcissism.

Thus, for the adolescent, the excessive corporeal practice has a double function: that of *I act, therefore I exist*, and one which is specific to each practice. The muscles swollen through weightlifting, display the prestige of the muscle and of a well-made body, represent the visualization of virility, a machismo of a body image as opposed to the defective one of the past. For the *tattooist*, the notch practiced on the body expresses the pain of the feeling and represents recognition of the self and of its image. But this jouissance and recognition of one's own body is not without mischief; the price is that the body that has become the object and is no longer the body of the subject. The symptomatic and fetishistic act, in effect, wanting to be an identitary substitute, through a sadistic passage to the act exerted on the body and/or the skin space favored by the narcissistic chasm of the body image and the ambiguity of instinctual emergence, leads the body to become both subject and object of itself.

In order to understand the genesis of the acting body, we consider, on the contrary, an action on the body and skin, carried out by another from birth, such as excessive packing or mummification of the baby. The infant who is imprisoned for several months, even years, in tightened linens, put at the margin of touch and movement, a passive recipient of the *mise at a distance* promoted by the anguish of the parents becomes a *mummifized* adolescent. This means that the image of the mummified skin and the rigidness of the body will be inhibitory defense mechanisms of the ego and the body. In fact, a doubling of imagos is installed: the body seen is not the "true" body; the *true* body is the fantasized body, virtualized. The adolescent confines his lived body in a virtual image, and hides it by means of theatrical clothing in another body - that of reality.

In the next three chapters, we will focus on the adolescent passage to the act manifested in the glory of the muscles of the *bodybuilder*, the imprinted skin of the *tattooist*, and finally the virtual body of the *mummifized* in order to demonstrate the doubling of imagos of the body: the hidden body, phantomatized, on the one hand, and the displayed body, aestheticized, through sculpture, drawing or art of clothing on the other, leading to a pathology of the corporeal narcissism.

Chapter 1

THE BUILT BODY

INTRODUCTION

"Before I had only empty skin, a nothing skin. I played sports. My body and me are one thing, we're the same thing. Me my body, my body me" [Interview, Tareck, 17 years old].

In the society of display, self-image is intended to be captivating. Fragile and ethereal women and thin and super muscular men want to be seen. Often, a comparison is made with these overworked images; the youth and those who are younger try to copy the models presented, dreaming, sometimes more than reasonably, to replace the model. To be seen, admired and applauded seems to be everyone's ultimate goal. This modeling of the ideal body can become symptomatic, even pathological.

In order to capture the gaze of the other and the others, some adolescents settle into a muscular escalation, becoming *bodybuilders* (excessively dependent on sports and later on anabolic steroids). What do we understand from this practice: Is it a passage to the act on the body which becomes the object of sadistic practice turned against the self? The compensation by the sculpture of the muscle, of a felt lack? The reinforcement of the muscle in place of penile erection?

"In the kingdom of triumphant virility for which the preferred use of body-organism, the appetence for corporeal control via muscular work comes to make up for the deficit of psychic interiorization and/or substitutes to the overflow of emotions [...]" [2: 241]. Yes, but why is this so and how do we understand the use of such a palliative? What image of his body does the adolescent have; which leads him towards the realization, through the physical act, of a central transformation? What does he want to change, by substituting the past body, which is seen as rejected, denied and hidden with the newly acquired corporeality? Who is this adolescent?

Our hypothesis takes into consideration the doubling of body imagos. It seems, in fact, that a defective archaic body image is substituted with a new image that is no less defective, and acts through a mutilative motivation, taking the body as an object, is at the origin of the dependence upon sports and anabolic steroids among adolescent bodybuilders. This corporeal archaism, acting as a narcissistic abdication, leads the bodybuilder to search into the mirror of the self for a new image that is over-invested of an Ego/body-ideal.

To implement this work, a population was selected according to specific criteria defining bodybuildism. There were semi-structured clinical interviews with 18 adolescent bodybuilders between the ages of 15 and 20 which supported our data. The administration of TAT to Sami (18 years old), a *bodybuilder* for 3 years and 2 months, and to Jenny (17 years old), a bodybuilder for 2 years and 7 months, serves as an illustration.

1. THE FINITENESS OF THE MIRROR AND THE OTHER PSYCHE

"Henceforth the image of the body-seen takes over the images of the body-lived. It is at the age of three and throughout our entire existence that the image of the body-seen imposes itself [...]" [3: 27].

The imaginary impression of the body begins with the corporeal sensations of the baby (maternal breast, environment, etc.) until the discovery of the image of his/her own body. This image of the body, based on the body schema - a neurological substrate- is charged with affectivity and the relational. It is built from memories, emotions, and the involvement of parents and of the significant Other. The meaning that the bodybuilder gives to his body, the gaze that he draws, and the way he speaks, is a fundamental articulation for the comprehension of the subject.

The lexical fields of interviews with adolescent bodybuilders first take hold of the body and its nudity: *"I like living with my muscles bare."* (Sami, 18 years old). The bodybuilder carries with him the exhibited nudity and is apprehended by it; *"I am my self when my body is bare"* (Nadyne, 20 years old). It seems that, to the contrary, the body gathers the gaze on itself. The body is what ensures the gaze.

The bodybuilder appears to be vigilant to the gaze of others. (The terms of the category Gaze: *to gaze, to see, to be seen, vision or invisible, hidden, etc.*, are used 24 times on average per interview). His identity and the feeling of existing pass through the gaze of the other upon his body, *"My body sees itself"* (Gilles, 16 years old), *"The gazes on my body, I adore that"* (Jenny, 17 years old).

By default of having been able to be unified in the psyche of his childhood, the bodybuilder attempts to unify the posed gazes of approval on his body. It is the seen body that is the body. *"I see myself seen"* (Alex, 18 years old).

Table 1. Lexical fields related to Bodybuildism - identified from interviews

Body and Gaze		Bad and Good Image	Space and Reparation	Mother	Father
Pain in the body	Be seen	Underestimate/ Esteem	Club	Abandonment	Absence
Biceps	Eyes	Lack of trust/	Space	Absence	Beauty
Body	Form	Trust	Running	Anger	Coldness
Chest	Gaze	Ugly/ Beauty	-----------------	Authority	Distance
Clothing	Invisibility	Puny/Strong	Amphetamines	Breach	Force
Muscle	Mirror	Fatigue/	Ephedrine	Coldness	Incapacity
Nudity	Presence	Seduction	Products (AS)	Detachment	Indifference
Torso	Sight	Depressive/	Proteins	Despotism	Laxity
Thorax	Vision	Assurance	Pill	Disaffection	Monstrosity
Weight		Illness/Healthy	Training 6/10h	Disenchantment	Perversion
				Disinterest	Violence
				Distance	Weakness
				Egoism	Wickedness
				Eroticization	
				Inattention	
				Indifference	
				Insensitivity	
				Misunderstanding	
				Narcissism	
				Negligence	
				Rejection	
				Seduction	
				Selfishness	
(444) 874(430)		802	317	820	373

Without that gaze, the feared fragmentation would appear. In the gaze of others, and in his own, the bodybuilder opposes his uniqueness to the multiplicity of the parts that compose it. In all the interviews, parts of the body are cited (*chest, muscle, biceps, etc.*) but it is when *he sees himself seen*, that he speaks of his body as an entity. His ego identifies with his image, his body, *"There is me now in the big mirror"* (Julien, 17 years old). Corporeal narcissism is identifiable because it is different from the image of other bodies: the body is therefore a unique model, original, irreplaceable. *"I live when I look at myself"* (Sami, 18 years old). This image having become the referrer of the Ego and its characteristics comfort the narcissism. *"It will not be me I will be someone else without my body"* (Jenny).

Once the body is built, it will be even less possible for the subject to stop the exercises and the consumption of AS out of fear that his body will be modified again and deconstructed into ugliness. The sportive act becomes a ritualization, which leads its adaptation to a continuous control of the image in the mirror.

For the author of *Écrits*, the mirror stage is formative of the function of the subject, the *I*. He previously spontaneously identified the other with himself through the process of introjection, and himself with the other through that of projection. At the end of the Lacanian jubilation experience, the child will recognize his Ego. The identification with the specular image provides the child with a sense of unity substituting for the fragmentary feeling of existing until then. For Julien and other bodybuilders, the feeling of jubilation appears only belatedly. This identification (*I*, said Julien) is not recognition, but misrecognition: the subject confuses himself with the image in the mirror. The identification is then narcissistic [3: 98]; surely the mirror stage structures the personality, but it is especially the definitive inscription, the finiteness of the subject in his biological body. Far from being jubilant, the child suffers from this symbolic castration, attempting to subjectify the unconscious image of himself in the reflected image [4]. If at a later stage, the child recognizes the image of otherness in an intersubjective dimension the bodybuilder on his own behalf is fixated on the image of narcissistic misrecognition: the Ego will become an image, and not the image, the image of me. *"I was nothing before my sport"* (Adel, 16 years old).

The salience of this bodybuilding lure allows an understanding of the rationalized reinterpretation of the constituent details of the body image by the Ego. The designation of the body captures the subject in a chain of signifiers. Everything happens as if the perceived body creates the ego and actualizes it through the gaze.

The child proves his unity, more in the parents' gaze and sayings, in others, than in his own image. The gaze is fundamental because it allows the identification with oneself by the specular image and the identification of the self through the image in the Other's gaze. Therefore, the specular image and the image in the gaze of the other will serve as models for the constitution of the subject.

"I had no mirror" (Gilles); *"I looked at myself, I did not recognize myself, I thought: this is not me"* (Amin, 17 years old); *"I had cast a curse, I was an ugly frog"* (Nadyne, 20 years old). The muscles that the bodybuilder so proudly exhibits are in fact a response to this feeling of not being seen or not having been seen, the same as not to be seen, not to be recognized by himself and not to be distinct, *"I do not think my father sees me"* (Bassam, 18 years old); *"I met my mom at times down the stairs, she took time to recognize me, I said: it's me[...]"* (Sami, 18 years old).

This is precisely the object relationship that led Dolto [5: 69] to define the unconscious image of the body as a relational-structure model. This picture is causal and built from the one reflected by the Other. This image combined and mixed, sometimes disparate and heteroclite, presents misfires, bad-builds, lacks, chasms. However accomplished the image, the young child realizes that others cannot access him other than by what he gives them to see, he "privileges the appearances and neglects his internal sensations. Henceforth, he will forget the inside to handle only the outside. The bitterness of disillusionment gives rise to the unconscious craftiness of a child who recuperates the specular image at the expense of his narcissism" [6: 27]. The adolescent bodybuilder is subtracted in a corporealized-idealized narcissism; the unity of *I* continues to be based, for him, on the narcissistic ideal.

Narcissus, in the waters of his gaze, is in love with himself. The ultimate search of the bodybuilder is the perpetual search of an externalized ego that has become an object rather than a subject. Of this object, the thing-body becomes the subject: *"My biceps, this is my brand, it's me"* (Amer, 18 years old); *"My body made me alive"* (Jenny, 17 years old).

The subjection of the Ego to the body image permits the observation of a narcissistic closure in the bodybuilder, an exclusive dependency on his muscular envelope invested in the self. The bodybuilder always doubles his body; there is in fact the invisible body, unrecognized, suffering, denied, the *"frog"* body of childhood, and the body/ego ideal that wants to be distinguished, particularized, object of gaze, but by returning, body-subject to which the ego identifies. *"This body makes me forget the body that I have never been"* (Bernard, 16 years old); *"My phantom body [...]"* (Tareck, 17 years old). The Ideal Ego must be searched for because the body has suffered from being nobody's body.

Unlike competitive athletes who submit their bodies to the goals of victory and records set, the feeling of wellbeing and beauty is primordial. Bodybuilding fans, however, live their bodies as an end, as the supreme means of perception for others and as beyond communication. Psychologically dependent on their corporeal fantasies, (what Pope et al., 2000, [7] call the *Adonis complex* and relate to psychosis), bodybuilders transform the imagery of a beautiful and powerful body, with a finality to which they may never arrive which induces the repetition.

In fact, the bodybuilder is faced with the limitations of his body and his performance capability. He therefore seeks to overcome them. In this fissure, the past body, the body hidden by the newness of the muscles, is the object of the suffering repetition, on which the overwhelmed ego exercises its aggression through sadism turned against oneself.

The pain inflicted by others has become the pain inflicted by oneself. It is this pain that leads to destroying oneself with anabolic steroids and to be flogged. *"These minor discomforts of amphetamines are nothing; they are only benefits* (good-fits)" (Tareck, 17 years old).

While the body of the sportive culturism is the narcissistic body, the ego ideal. The bodybuilder, who has two bodies, has no body. The one denied is the child whose body was forgotten. The other, proclaimed, is that of the dethroned ego because it is corporealized.

The body/ego is invested in its capacity to produce, to manufacture even more muscle, thereby relegating into forgetfulness the slender and infantile body. Production that relates back to an reified ego *(object, sculpture)*; to the permanent lure that is established between the production and the quality of the body/ego that can be exhibited, like a factory that calculates its production on the quality of materials *(AS, training, hours of musculature, pills, etc.)*. The ultimate irony in building his body/ego is that the bodybuilder destroys the I/subject through castrating auto-mutilation.

Everything comes down to the made body. Body/ego exalted but sacrificed body; split body.

In the lexical fields of interviews (table) the mother appears as not containing, but she is unstable in her relation to the child; sometimes rejecting and indifferent, sometimes phallic but especially narcissistic and eroticizing; while the father seems weak, violent and powerless. How do we understand the recourse to the bodybuilder act in this family functioning?

The recreating gaze held on the body is primarily that of the mother. Winnicott [8] speaks of a house for the psyche in the body through the structuring illusion of the good enough mother. The indifferent mother, by contrast, prevents the differentiation from occurring and will create in her child a precocious narcissistic disinvestment. *"When I was little, I did not like myself. [...] Mom was afraid to touch me, the maid gave me the bath"* (Sami, 18 years old); *"Mom doesn't know the color of my eyes [...], I think she doesn't see me"* (Nadyne, 20 years old). The bodybuilder defends himself against the expressionless void in the maternal gaze, never ceasing to detail the reflection of his muscles in the mirror turned into a *psyche*.

Anzieu [9] considers that the skin-ego shores upon the various functions of the skin: a function of containment, of limits, of inscription of traces, of communication. The mother, by correctly interpreting and ensuring the needs of her baby, constructs an envelope of wellbeing, and supports the secure illusion of double narcissism - omnipotence and omniscience. Without this magical illusion, the child does not inscribe: *"I was like a bag with something in it"* (Amin, 17 years old).

By her non-acceptance, the *rejecting* mother has neglected the child's body and his psychic integration. Paradoxically, the child lacking the omnipotent illusion, does not structure his limits. So, as soon as possible, the person without magical illusion and without boundaries will have recourse to sports and SA as substitutes for his mother's insufficiently containing arms, a practice giving him an omnipotent satisfaction, but he is unable to limit it, searching in his dependency more and more every day.

The bodybuilding club becomes a place of containment: *"The club welcomes me"* (Nadyne); *"I am good at the club"* (Alex, 18 years old); a feeling of well-being is established that the mother could not provide, the feeling of the person, the sense of being: *"When I started going to the club, I knew that I was someone who I was in care"* (Bernard, 16 years old) and a space in which to establish the conditions of being alone and being with others: *"At the club we're together, and each one, and I like it"* (Bassam, 17); *"Nobody invaded me, yet we are many"* (Amer, 18 years old). The feeling of strangeness falls: *"I do not know the others, except one or two, but I know that we are the same"* (Tareck, 17 years old).

This *indifferent* mother prevents the differentiation from occurring and creates in her child an early narcissistic disinvestment. *"When I was little, I did not like myself. I do not even know if someone loved me."* The narcissistic disinvestment of the Ego, as an object of the Id, leads to the loss of its objectal quality. The Ego that is prematurely solicited will develop alarming conducts, representatives of the death instinct, in their neutralization function, even mortification of excitement. A Winnicottian false self is constructed. *"I asked for nothing. I did not cry"* (Bernard, 16 years old). Later, a false body appears, mortifying the ego.

But this *narcissistic* mother is occupied only with her beauty, and the child, seeing his mother preferring her own body, will look at his. By a subtle identification with the aggressor, the body develops; it rivals that of the mother. From poorly built, it becomes muscular, imposing, sculpted. The body wants to be recognized by the mother; from being invisible it becomes visible, swollen and important. The body wants to seduce the blind mother; from being colorless, it becomes beautiful, seductive, and phallic. *"I like to show her I'm more beautiful than her"* (Amer).

The mother is, moreover, *seductive*. The incestuous leads to the fantasmic impasse and provokes a stunning thought along with the excitement, and bars the access to individuation. The child who is defenseless because of his age and of his situation no longer understands the conjugation of rejection and seduction, *"She made me sleep next to her the night I was her favorite [...], during the day she forgot me, I no longer existed"* (Alex). The oscillation between the under-containment and maternal erotic over-containment is in rapport with confusional and incestuous lived experiences. This oscillation characterizes the paradoxical narcissistic position that is presented as a defense against the anguishes of separation and union. The mother establishes links of influence in the proximity with her child, and then brutally puts him at a distance, leaving him unprotected. If the analysis on violence aims at the appropriation of the object for its destruction, the anaclisis on of the corporeal body of the bodybuilder, in the opposition hate-love is of advantage in the appropriation of the object by attraction and admiration in order to fight against the catastrophic anguishes of collapse and the recourse to violence.

In summary, the mother of the bodybuilder is an unstable mother. When talking of instability it situates the term within its structural value: within its cleaving dimension. It is not of the ambivalent position of *I love you but leave me in peace*, or *I love you and I hate you*, but of what we call an *unstable splitter position*, which is *come in to my bed and you doesn't exist*. Ambivalence creates the conditions that lead to a search of the univocal, beyond hate; cleaving instability, however, it leads only to a doubling of positions.

The father appears powerful and defective, strong and weak, violent and permissive. In fact *"He made his life outside the house and does not take care of us"* (Bassam). *"Everyone loves dad because he helps them, but at home we hate him"* (Nadyne). *"People say that Dad is strong, but I find him weak"* (Gilles). Unstable Imago leaves the adolescent in a distressed state: *"I do not know what to do with him, what to say to him"* (Sami). However, it is the image of the castrating father who dominates, *"Dad is beautiful, he pleases, but with my muscles I will be more handsome than him."* The lack of the penis anguishes the child, *"Dad said, you are beast and muscular. Yet when the body is beautiful one is afraid of nothing"* (Gilles, 16 years old). The adolescent revolts: his father can be found on the path of his fantasies, of his desires, of his power, of his muscular erection. The father is the castrator, but recognizable.

Unable to face the castration, the bodybuilder calls for compensatory mechanisms; his muscles in erection want to make him believe in his erectile power. The false semblance of this second lure leads to the addictive repetition: *"If I feel a little soft, I go to the club"* (Bassam, 17 years old); *"I am a sportsman, of what am I afraid"* (Tareck). From the workout, to food, to the multiplicity of hours of training, to stronger and stronger steroids, the chain of dependency is installed, locking the adolescent into a circle of illusions. He believes he will no longer fear his anguish, but in fact he flees it; the avoidance and denial of the castrating apprehension takes place.

Powerless to face castration, the "act of breakup between the mother and the child, which slices the imaginary of its narcissistic link" [10: 140], the bodybuilder substitutes it with a marking of the body. Indeed, rejected, humiliated, and unrecognized by one's own, a stranger to himself and others, the child, through reparation and compensation mechanisms, tries to give himself an identity: sports becomes a sign, a mark of recognition by replacing the deficient father. *"I needed my father, but he was not there"* (Sami); *"My father gave me nothing, I learned nothing"* (Gilles); *"If he could put me up for adoption by anyone, he would have been happy"* (Bassam); *"[...] neither father nor mother, now I do sports"* (Mario, 16 years old).

The *castrating and phallic* maternal imago who interdicts the access to the symbolic field of the father is omnipresent for the young bodybuilder. Implacable, cold, despotic and blind to the welfare of the child, she believes herself omnipotent.

The child believes in her and for him she is the bearer of the phallus. By the bodybuilding, the muscular erection, the adolescent gives himself an attribute of power, *"My muscles make me strong"* (Bassam) and *"I frighten my mom with my biceps"* (Tareck). The built body becomes the phallic substitute for the mother. The muscles, acting as fetish, come to mask the anguished representation of the archaic castration. The possession of the muscle thus ensures the means to triumph over the terrible maternal imago, *"She will see in a few months how my muscles are strong"* (Gilles).

Only the paternal metaphor can allow the mother to be the subject of the deprivation and a place of lack. The father, an "agent of the humanizing symbolic cutting" [11: 246], allows the passage to the significant world. By contrast, the eventual vice of the cut mother/child can be translated through the foreclosure of that signifier. But the importance that the mother gives to the father's word will condition the anchor of the paternal function in each subject.

The mother of the bodybuilder is a mediocre mediator; the father in her eyes is *"incapable"* (Ghaleb 18 years old); *"nosy"* (Gilles 16 years old); *"unsatisfied"* (Mario 16); *"a monster"* (Sami 18 years); *"an adulterer"* (Hosni 17 years); *"a violent aggressor"* (Bernard, 16 years old); *"a pervert"* (Jenny, 17 years old); *etc.* "The Father, with the body envied by the son, seems to the mother's eyes both impotent and sexually violent. But in the eyes of the son, he is an adulterer with ambiguous sexuality: *"Dad has relationships outside, but perhaps with men."* (Bassam, 17 years); *"I think daddy is bisexual"* (Nadyne); *"Dad's adventures outside the home, and many, even if mom says he is not satisfied in sex"* (Sami).

How then can the bodybuilder, with *an incapable or violent* father, a father who is the object of a weakened maternal mediation, pretend to the symbolic castration? In addition, the identificatory imago relative to the sexuality of the father is floating and the adolescent seems undecided as to how to determine it.

The homosexuality of the father seems fairly present leaving the son bewildered in the accomplishment of the identificatory processes of his sexuality: To please the father, would it require that he take a feminine attitude? Gilles is the only subject in the study to say clearly *"I'm gay"*; the other subjects, even when asked directly about their sexuality, respond ambiguously: *"I should try"* (Sami); *"I think I like it"* (Nadyne); *"No I am I mean I'm not, but I do not know if it's good to be"* (Hosni); *"I do not know"* (Bassam).

The bodybuilder, in fact, has not accomplished but only approximated one or more of the conditions for *humanization*. The bodybuilder with an unstable mother and a father with contestable sexuality attempts to rediscover a significant other. He seeks to move away from an identificatory image with the mother without a penis (the clitoris equivalent to being without muscles), but the father is defective. Identificatory processes could not be accomplished and he finds in the body that becomes the Ego-ideal, a repetitive mechanism that is compensatory to castration.

"I had no choice, I had to die, or I wanted to live, I chose sport to live, and I have started" (Sami). The culturist passage to the act, which is characterized by a triple addiction, is, in fact, an adolescent aggressive act turned against oneself.

It is the object relations that will allow an awareness of pubertal experiences. At this age a narcissistic reorganization, that permits the internalization of body modifications and access to the changes in object relations, is inscribed. The bad is projected or else it is split. Green [11: 53-60] insists on the splitting of the ego of the subject, that in order to maintain its cohesion it refuses to see itself as bad. The object is ex-corporated. From this perspective, the castration would be related to the disinvestment of a partial object, invested with a narcissistic libido. However, this process would allow the investment of total objects that provide a narcissistic safeguard. The object is then used for narcissistic means; Eros becomes a source of survival and unbinding and of destruction of the object. Survival is the death of the other. This way the aggressive adolescent conserves the link with the libido [12: 481-502] by making use of violence that aims for an assertion of an integrated individual ego in an attempt to safeguard his ego through an illusory omnipotence. This violence of the safeguard, of the omnipotence manifested through the body, the bodybuilder turns it against himself.

The relation of strangeness with his body puts into question the identity of the future bodybuilder. The child is devalued, and in response to his anguishes of loss and to his defective narcissism, he will resort to splitting and the doubling of imagos of his corporeality in order to avoid confrontation with the depressive position; and he thus finds himself in a narcissistic pathology: *"I have suffered a lot in starting sport, I have cried, I have struggled. [...]. I have suffered a lot when I was a frog [...]"* (Nadyne). The unintegrated body modifications; the bodybuilder will accomplish them; he becomes actant and actor of his modifications but also excessively dependent on sports and AS. Tareck used to hide under the table when he was a child in order to become invisible and to avoid parental abuse and humiliating words targeted at his shriveled body. Today, it is under the muscles of his body that he hides his puny body.

Adolescence assumes, for the child of the discredited and humiliated body, a value of engulfment in which individuation is confronted with the risk of destruction threatening both the subject and object. The unabsorbed preoedipal violence, conjoint to libidinal aggressiveness, leads the adolescent to a passage to a bodybuildism act that becomes not only a survival mechanism, but a mortifying survival. Sexuality is lived in an aleatory way,

"Now with my body, I can turn the girls' head" (Gilles 16 years old); *"It shocks you if I say I'm gay since I started my sport"* (Sami); *"I do not care who my sexual partner of the moment is, I have my sport!"* (Hosni, 17 years old). *"Without sports there is no sexuality",* they all proclaim, albeit *"sex is secondary, sport comes first,"* as Alex expresses it very succinctly.

The maternal under-containment and the laxity of the father present sequels on diverse levels: in the processes of integration of the ego and the formation of the false self, on the level of the thought and the acquisition of symbolic, as well as at the behavioral level through the creation of behavioral automatism. The bodybuilder has pain at the body-ego so, through a mechanism of pathological repetition, he will endeavor by muscular sculpture to recover this unsatisfactory integration of the image.

The body is then inscribed in the register of the physical and becomes a veritable body-machine destined for performance and exploitation. Intensive training, constantly repeated, will lead the bodybuilder to forge an ideal body, meeting the requirements of its practice under the primacy of perceptible beauty. This modeling of the body required an overinvestment of the muscular register at the expense of the psychical sphere. But the hidden, invisible body, the body of the self, remains, whatever it does different from the forged body, forced in the mirror.

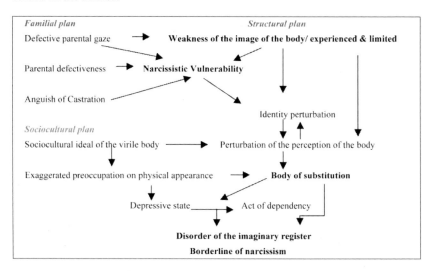

Graph 1. Schema of the action of diverse psychological and socio-anthropological factors in the etiology of Bodybuildism.

Therefore, the bodybuilding passage to the act is a form of language, a substitute for the lack, a means of identity defense, an illusory recognition of the ego through the body by an adolescent struggling with himself. Bodybuildism is a new pathology of the imaginary.

2. TWO ADOLESCENTS AND THEIR BODY

"To be systematically losing does not stop him, but rather bases him, in his individual myth and longing to be magnificent. [...]. He is the royal waste of the Other. Triumphant victim returns to him the palm of martyrdom. [...]. And he becomes a heroic witness of the Passion of castration" [13: 39].

2.1. Sami

Sami, 18, has been practicing bodybuilding since the age of 15 years and currently does 6 hours of daily physical education, with steroid consumption that began last year. He is pursuing technical studies in acoustics, which downgrades him in relation to his wealthy parents (a surgeon father and an interior designer mother). He aspires to become a CEO and describes himself as someone who is *"misunderstood and lonely."* He has only bad memories from his childhood; he was *"ugly and shy"* and did not please *"even his mother."* he cried alone in his room. He contemplated suicide, but accidentally turned to physical culturism, where he found *"a reason to live."* The only person that mattered to him and to whom he mattered was his elder sister of three years, Sarah.

During the administration of the tests, under his apparent annoyed air, Sami was anxious; (he played with his fingers, rubbed his chin, moved continuously in his chair, etc.).

The projected perception that the adolescent has of himself reveals a narcissistic problematic (c. 1: *This has nothing to do with the perfection of the body ...why did you give me this picture?*). An intrapsychic conflict appears to be playing on the interpersonal stage. Infatuated with his body, his anguish before the card appears through denegation and a call to the clinician. (*A boy distracted by an instrument, a guitar, it may be possible that he is thinking about how it was made; he is probably thinking of the most perfect way to play or to produce a stylized sound*).

The representations of action associated with emotional states reflect Sami's affective and emotional liability. The search for compensatory idealization is marked by qualifiers attached to the perceptual (*perfection of the body, perfect manner, and stylized sound*).

The idealization of self-representation reappears (c. 6BM: *[...] I am intelligent, with all modesty...*), but is associated, again, with a strongly present narcissistic failure, and a feeling of guilt: (... *If someone is not intelligent, he does not understand this picture. The servants of a wealthy family! This is the maid, seen through her clothes. And this young man who wears a uniform must be the driver. It seems that they were reprimanded, a reprimand like no other, it is seen on his face, while for her, she is wretched. It is quite possible that they have committed a serious offense for which they are being rebuked*). Is it not the brother and sister who are abused, and their rich parents who make them feel guilty? The mother/son relationship in the card is not recognized. It is presented in a context of inferiority, humiliation and guilt, *"We the children passed in second. Sometimes, when we were extremely small, mom forgot to pick us up from school. Sarah held my hand, but I was still afraid. When she finally arrived, she rebuked us, saying that she was late because of us."* Sami does not dare to face the guilt that comes from the negative emotions that he feels towards his mother and seeks to justify her persecuting and castrating attitude, *"She was never satisfied with me. [...]. She only taught me criticism."*

The wounded narcissism is accompanied by a problematic of loss and abandonment (c.13B: *Poor boy! Your images become tragic. This poor boy lost his parents*); but also of archaic powerlessness and castration (*because the absence of light behind shows that this boy has no back, without help, there is nobody to protect him in this life. He is barefoot, has a melancholic appearance, abandoned, uprooted*). Sami, uprooted, feels he no longer belongs to his environment and declares with bitterness: *"My parents are ashamed of me and think I'm a ruffian."* The only place where he feels comfortable, where he feels at home, without judgment and without criticism, is his club: *"This is where I am myself [...]. The club is my home. [...]. I feel comfortable, like everyone else."*

The relationship to the archaic maternal imago appears to be a source of pathology (c. 11: *This is a fortress, there is a door, and it is a fortress on the water. This bridge is dangerous and below is nothingness; it is dark because of a severe storm, a man fled on the bridge. He drags cerberuses behind him*). The young man introduces into the card bizarre and non-existent characters, and his story is rich in disorganized and altered elements reflecting the presence of a pregenital problematics.

As for the general emotional tone of the interview, we note anger and anguish in the mother/child relationship. *"With mom we did not know how to act. White or black, it was random."* The absence of nuances reflect the anguish of the child in his relations with his unstable, splitter mother; anguish even stronger because it seems undetermined.

The father, even more than the mother, is present/absent (c. 7BM: *Whoever made these images, did he plagiarize or invent them? There is an old man and a young man. The old man tries to talk to the young man to guide him, reason with him or help him. I personally see it from two perspectives: 1. The young man is the son of the old man because sadness is spread on his face, he was at fault and the old man said: therefore understand, you must be this and that, etc. etc.. 2. or when the old man realized that the young man had had enough of him ... He wears a suit and the figure of the old man looks sad*). The massiveness of obvious processes - the direct entry into expression, the call to the clinician, the important intra-narration silence, the contrasted representation, the reaction formation, the verbal caution, the hesitation between two versions, the blurred discourse, the evocation of a bad object, the insistence on the faces, the false perception, the discourse disturbance, the loss of logical causality, and the emergence of a disordered and altered projection - reveals the presence of a strong father-son conflict. The son is represented in an inferior position in relation to the superegoic and disapproving paternal imago, which reveals a castration and repressed aggression, *"Dad is ugly, [...] I was afraid of dad [...] he is a selfish and insignificant man"* says the adolescent, projecting a doubled imago of the father, and involving again the body in a compensatory movement that is not openly expressed. Sami is beautiful and muscular, and this is his only victory against the castrating father.

The desire to murder the father is justified by the son. (c. 8BM: *A man is dead, killed ... This young man is an artist, a poet who told about her father, a fighter who resisted was shot at, another was wounded and then a third man came to help*).

The evocation of a murder followed by an interpretation then a loss of logical causality through reaction formation, identificatory projection and a flood of expressions, relate to an aggressive theme and a theme of castration, show a repressed aggressive drive against a powerful masculine imago that can represent the father. The disorganized speech and the massiveness of the primary processes reveal the intensity of the conflict, which appears without a process of avoidance.

The Oedipal problematic is present. Sami acknowledges the sexual impulses, aggressive and fatal - (c. 13MF: *There is a sick and naked woman, she is covered with a sheet, at her side there is a young doctor, his treatment has failed and the woman died. One can also see a sexual relationship between this young man and this woman. He has silenced his desire, and she remained asleep, and so he tries to leave*) - however the tonality is labile. Indeed, the subdivision of the narration into two interpretations permitting the emergence of a splitting, equivalent to the reaction formation and avoidance announces the projection of a powerless masculine image, incapable, and afraid of female sexual desire, *"Mom, the way she thinks is grave. [...] I try to keep myself far from her."*

While the family dysfunction is clearly apparent in the interview, *"My father never had time for us, he was very busy with his patients, [...] he was here on Sunday, but he was cold [...]. We would have preferred that they'd argue, it would have given us some warmth."* There is icy coldness for the child which is a sign of unresolved conflicts. The mother, on the other hand, is rather whimsical and unstable *"Sometimes she scolded us and punished us, sometimes she would let us do as we pleased, [...] the way she thinks is really strange, nothing is clear."* The parents intervened inappropriately with their children, imposing limits, either strict or poorly defined. Most of the time, the child's reaction was characterized by non-adherence and submission *"My sister and I understood nothing, but we obeyed."* The incapacity of the subject to address the affect (c. 1, 6BM, 11, 19) after a clear inhibition, and the rechewing and hesitation prompted by these cards, underline the presence of this conflict.

The parental couple appears to be anguished (c.10: *A married couple, a man and a woman hug, but the woman said goodbye because the man will die soon*). The perception of the allied couple is intolerable, and for the second time, Sami kills the father. The ambivalence in the representation of the couple and the emergence of morbid elements refer to archaic elements of persecution. Separation, loss and an aggressive drive are all detected. We find this intolerance again in the interview: *"I say my parents, but there is no father or mother or couple, neither parents nor children."*

The family dynamic is organized around reactions that make the process of individuation and adaptation difficult. This includes the disengagement of the father, the inappropriate maternal investment and neglect, the several inappropriate basic educational acts (severe punishment, verbal abuse, seclusion, eroticization ...), and consequent emotional states (sadness, anguish, depression).

The refusal tendency points out an inability to integrate his own interiority, (c. 16: *Nothing comes to mind. I do not talk much about myself, I don't express myself, after this thing what are you going to show me?*); Sami remains glued to the external image of his body, and refuses to look any further. The insistence on the limits and contours of the sensory qualities and of the percept in all the cards shows his dependence on external objects put forward to palliate for the deficiencies of internal objects (parental superego and self-identity). This splitting strongly existing is indicative of an experience with a persecutory archaic maternal object. As for the misperception, the call to the clinician and the personal reference all announce insurmountable castration anguish. The doubling of imagos also appears in the reflections between the unloved and ungazed child and the beautiful adolescent in the mirror, links are not established.

The young man is bogged down in the archaic stages of development. His narcissism is threatened by a phobogenic relation with an unstable mother and a paradoxically absent and frightening father. A fragile ego and non-incorporated superego conjure up a picture, which is not very encouraging of a dependent personality, who tries to fill in the gaps by resorting to the act.

2.2. Jenny

Jenny, who is 16 years and 11 months old, is very tall and very muscular. She began practicing sports to excess at the age of 14 years and 4 months, and three months ago she started taking anabolic steroids. She is the eldest daughter of a family of three children (two girls and a boy). The boy is the youngest and the sweetheart of the family. She says that her mother is depressed, that she suffered from baby blues at her birth, and that she did not have time to care for her or the other children. Jenny left school and is preparing for a career in hair care. Her technical studies leave her enough free time to practice bodybuilding (5 hours per day and 6 to 8 hours on both weekend days). She thinks that when she was little, she was shy, thinking that *"life is hard [...] is something frightening,"* but she is *"afraid of nothing since I do sports."* Jenny's father is employed in a major juice factory and the mother is a cook in a famous fast food restaurant. Jenny has always dreamed of becoming a football champion. Her expression is transformed when she talks about her brother and sister; the bond that she has with them *"allows her to survive."* The children seem to delight in complicity against their parents: *"We tell them nothing about what we do, but between us we always know*

[...]." There is a sensitive narcissistic conflict between the two sisters; the little one seeks to imitate the eldest and finds a happy conclusion. *"My sister gets on my nerves sometimes, but I have only her. So I agreed to give her my things. She wants to play sports at the club, but I do not know if I should allow it."*

Jenny has a soft voice. She responds to the interview and pictures of the test, without apparent emotion in words and tone. But tension can be seen on her face contorted with effort, and her eloquent gestures take the role of words and express her distress.

The interview with Jenny reported a significant level of marital conflict and family dysfunction, specifically in the relationship with the mother, and the presence of unresolved conflicts within the family seems probable. This conflict takes on an important magnitude at home *"we are all concerned [...]. They argue [...]. Mom understands nothing [...]."* The adolescent is trying to hide the anguish which assails her to the evocation of these conflicts. She defends herself with manic reactions to card 4: she first tries a smile, then laughs strongly while wiping her eyes and begins her story with a marital conflict whose motive is not specified: (c. 4: *There is a man walking towards the faraway, he is angry, his wife is afraid, and she came to support him, but he kept walking, and he did not answer her calls ... then ... they walked together*). The problematic evokes Jenny's inability to express and to confess an aggression in the couple's life, despite the argued quarrel: The wife of the background is scotomized and the story remains undetermined. However, separation anguish is present and detected in the reaction of the female character who feels the fear of remoteness.

The feeling of isolation is strongly sensed and the adolescent suffers from it: (c. 13B: *There is a man who is angry or sad, he has nothing to eat. He suffers from something in his heart. People have or buy food, and sometimes they throw it, but nobody comes to give it to him*). Once again, sadness and anger are present in her speech, she who *"tries to never get angry,"* and are associated with a state of poverty and marginalization. The absence of solicitude from others is a source of melancholic affect, but Jenny seems unable to accept it. She populates her story with characters and objects in order to drown her isolation anguish in the movement between possessiveness and withdrawal. *"When I'm at the club, I do not talk to people, only to the coach, but I know that everyone is there, and we are all, all at the club."* Loneliness is in fact a lack of containment, which she considers as belonging and recognition, and the club gives Jenny this belonging, which seems to be universal to her.

The maternal imago is demanding and forbidding. (c. 5: Uh ... *Look at what it is: there is a woman who was sleeping and woke up, she glanced around her, she was surprised ... because there was a dog and before she slept, everything was broken and a complete mess, and now everything is clean, and the person who put everything in order is her daughter*). Faced with this superegoic picture, Jenny experiences ambivalence; she fears her mother and dreads losing her love. If ambivalence does not appear at the level of affect, it appears at the level of contrasting representations (disorder/order). To be at a certain distance of the scene, the adolescent introduces the character of the dog whose entrance into the scene is a sign of the disorganization of identity reference. The instability of the mother disrupts, indeed, the girl loses her defensive mechanisms and isolates herself: *"Mom is sometimes quiet, but other times, she changes, and I don't know what to do when she shouts [...]. Sometimes, she tears my clothes, and I have nothing to put on, I lock myself in the bathroom."*

The idea of *"breaking things"* takes the form of rumination in Jenny's discourse during which she recalls, for example, the following: *"I must have been one or two years old, I did not know, my mom tied me up with a rope in the bed so I do not break things in the house. It's my grandfather (paternal) who prohibited her from doing so."* The passivity and obedience of Jenny can leave room for rebellion, anger and insubordination. *"I do not obey her as before."* We find, in the card 7GF, the mother/daughter conflict: but here we witness the victory, otherwise effective at least as a fantasmatic of the girl on the mother: (*There is a woman and her daughter, and the daughter has a cat, but her mom does not like cats. When the mother saw the kitten, she told her daughter: "Put it out," but the girl did not obey, and she cried. "Sit down!" The daughter was angry and the mother got mad and also slapped her... and the cat stayed*). Jenny begins her story by introducing characters and by making a false perception (baby/cat) and uses the representation of contrasting emotions between the mother and the daughter. There is use of denegation and an action associated with an emotional state of refusal and anger, then of expulsion and an action associated with an emotional state of sadness and disobedience, and finally an undoing of the subject of injunction. The mother-daughter conflicting ambivalence provokes a large number of mechanisms. The adolescent seeks to impose herself by defying her mother by opposing her wishes and orders. The story ends with the decision of the child to impose her will onto her mother. In other words, the rebellion is the center of the real mother-daughter conflict, and Jenny is always looking to score a victory, which means to defeat the maternal authority. There are signs of manipulation and emotional blackmail, but also formation of opposition and the refusal of identification and of feminine identity: *"I can have muscle and I do not need my mom's lipstick."*

However, if the adolescent attempts rebellion, the little girl is totally terrified of the mother. (c.11: *Change it for me please, it is scaring me.... What is it? I see nothing ... There is a lion and a..., what is its name? A flying crocodile. They attack each other ferociously. But something breaks and they die together*). This card is a source of dread for the adolescent. Her story is phallic, aggressive and morbid. The latent solicitations revive archaic mortiferous and persecutory fantasies: the devouring nature (lion) of the maternal imago is underlying, and the struggle for survival revealed through breaking the terror of fragmentation.

We grasp the same mortiferous fantasies in card 19. (c.19: *Oufff ... There is an ice house and people inside. There are also thieves who are hiding. No? No, impossible, one of the robbers stood up to explode the house. He made it explode and all the inhabitants died*). Jenny begins her story with an objection; the card makes her feel uncomfortable. The aggressive theme reflects the fear of the debacle: the house represents the ego of the young girl, an ego about to explode and disappear, a persecuted ego threatened by fragmentation, an ego that *"thieves"* can invade.

The management of the interior/exterior seems to be difficult, and Jenny is unable to project herself onto the whiteness of the paper (c.16: *(smile). White! You're lying to me, you're giving me an empty paper ... when I'll go to the club, we'll do sports together*). Jenny laughs and then makes a call to the clinician before which she presents herself as the victim of a lie, and finally evokes a bad object *(empty)* and passes to a reference stuck to external reality. The narcissistic fragility appears strongly through the victimizing position she takes, *"I think a lot of bad guys are around us,"* she says. In fact, the adolescent takes refuge in the external reality in an attempt to bypass her internal void.

The feeling of void pursues the girl, *"I always feel a void in my stomach; before, I used to eat, but it did not stop; now, I go to the club and it gets better."* The club to the adolescent represents the containment that she has not known in her mother's arms. *"In the children's playroom and sports area, there is a lovely swing, before I leave the club, I go to sit on the swing, to rock myself gently,"* as a tender lullaby that she has not known in her mother's arms, in which she has only known a *"void."*

Vacuity is at work as of the first card of TAT: (c. 1: *What is it? What's this boy's name? I do not know if he has a name. There beside him is a musical instrument. He is sitting, bored, he is alone, he needs money to buy food*). Interrogation and negation follow and reveal Jenny's disturbance. The problematic of castration is avoided through denegation. The phallic object is perceived without being named; however, she seeks to name the boy and the problematic of recognition and identity is evident and that of solitude is recognized.

The adolescent has the tendency to fill the lack with food, which once again expresses a feeling of lack of affection: castration and loneliness are both generators of the feeling of vacuity.

The void is also linked to a sense of morbidity and an experience of loss (c. 3BM: *I see nothing! What is it! There is a dead person in the coffin. It is the husband ... This woman has lost her husband and she came to see him, she started crying, she knelt on the floor and laid her head on the coffin. She has nothing*). The call to the clinician and the refusal tendency, the denegation followed by the perception of a deteriorated object and by the evocation of a bad object (death), as well as the rechewing, put in evidence the anguish of Jenny: having nothing, being nothing, being dead.

Experiencing love is one of Jenny's "*major concerns,*" and sexuality is hitherto repressed. The strong feeling of distress experienced in the previous card extends to this one and takes the form of inhibition: (c. 12BG: *There are trees, flowers and a boat ... but ... a girl is sleeping on the boat − laughs*). Jenny describes the landscape by focusing on details but in a limited manner. There is therefore the necessity to ask her some questions. She introduces a character that is not in the picture and she bursts out laughing. The adolescent remains stuck to external reality using a manic defense mechanism. Her perception is clearly eroticized.

Despite the back/forth movement between the instinctual expression and defense, Jenny eroticizes the couple's relationship: (c. 10: *What is this? There is a woman and a man dancing together who love each other dearly. Then the Mr. kisses her but not on her mouth, she leaned her head and he felt her smell and they danced*). Although the desire is thwarted by defense, this is a story of tenderness and sexual desire. The representation of the allied couple in love is recognized by the adolescent. Her sexuality, thin-skinned, is sensorialized by the movement of dance and the sensuality of smell.

The Oedipal triangulation is a creator of conflict for Jenny: (c. 2: *What is it? A seaside? I do not know. What is a statue? There is a statue, a sailboat near the sea, there is someone who is driving a horse and there is a young woman holding a book while she walks. Married? No, they are neighbors*). The massiveness of these processes - the call to the clinician, the tendency towards refusal, denegation, framing, hesitation between two different interpretations, anonymity of characters and the isolation between representations - as well as the wide range of defensive mechanisms -, undoing, denegation, sculpturing of the character of the mother and isolation between the man and the woman - are indicators of the presence of the conflict; the oedipal triangulation is quasi recognized and the oedipal conflict is apparent, but not resolved.

However, the problematic of card 6GF indicates a confusion of ages (*Who are they? Did you get them out of the movies? There is a woman and a man, who are divorced, and the girl says, "Fortunately, I am divorced, he treated me so badly." The man hears her and says, "Why do you say that?" She was surprised and said, "For no reason." He said: "Oh!" He thought about getting back with her, and at the end, they did get back together, and he did not beat her or rebuke her anymore*). The presence of contrasting representations reveals ambivalence between desire and defense. In other words, the girl cannot assume her feminine identity in the face of a seductive or desired male image, or an object of desire. This indicates a lack of self-esteem and a narcissistic fragility, and also presents a question mark on the quality of the relationship with the father and on the fate of sexualized identity. In fact, Jenny's relations with her father are disappointing to the adolescent who describes her father as sometimes absent, and sometimes an erotic and stressing agent; to her, he is an unstable, capricious, and difficult person. *"No one is to his liking, as if he is better [...]. We all feel uncomfortable when he walks around in his boxer shorts, he should be dressed. [...]. He thinks he is the center of the world."*

The denial of sexuality and of the concomitant conflict leads the adolescent to a disorder of identifications; (c.9GF: *A boy, yes it's a girl, she arranges her clothes and spreads them on the bed. What is it? She sees another girl running away, because she is afraid. A man is going to kill her because she has stolen something*). The apparent instability of identifications in the card, and the action associated with an emotional state of fear leaning towards persecution by a man who does not figure in the image, reflect a problem of identity in an oedipal, sexual and erotic context. The emphasis is placed on the corporeal acting and on persecution; in a latent eroticized movement (*she stole something*) susceptible to lead to fantasies (*going to kill her*), related to the reaction of the mother mortified by the theft.

The bed and the man with the dagger might reveal a violent sexual scene in the experience of the adolescent, as might such expressions in the interview: *"I protect my sister against men, she could be raped [...], men are like animals*

[...] These things (sex) are of savagery [...]," are rather eloquent and revealing of Jenny's ideas on and fears of sexuality. However, they remain ambiguous as the adolescent categorically refused to answer questions about possible sexual abuse: *"You have wrong and bad ideas, do not ask me this question anymore."* In summary, Jenny suffers from an incoherent family structure, with a lax father in relation to the laws, a rejecting, aggressive and unstable mother; all the while her fraternal links are a source of support and understanding.

The introduction of characters that are not shown in the picture demonstrates the adolescent's imaginary potential, but it also shows the ability to withdraw from external reality. To the young girl, populating the scene avoids the rise of an anguish of void and abandonment which sow in her the dread. This void *"in the stomach"* is linked to death, and to a food filling-in mechanism first then sports, which give her a feeling of safety, not only through the sport itself but also through a sense of containment that she grants to the club. The Oedipal conflict is initiated but not resolved. There is an inability in the young girl to assume her feminine identity against a penile masculine frightening image. However, we note the presence of the fantasy of seduction and the image of the allied and loving couple that makes Jenny dream. The inhibition of Jenny is evidence of the apparent neutralization of affect. The widely used anonymity of the characters allows the avoidance of the underlying anguish arising from the recognition of the protagonists of the conflict and the camouflage of guilt and aggression. It highlights the difficulty of tracking the identity of the young girl. The insistence on limits and contours reflect Jenny's effort to delineate the inside from the outside, involving a narcissistic fragility of the Ego and her inability to be autonomous.

The unitary representation of the image of the self and interiorization are missing in the girl, whose vulnerable ego is subject to manic manifestations. The hyper-instability of identifications or the oscillation between several identificatory positions reflects a mood disorder. Thus, the adolescent seeks to occupy all roles at once in order to avoid losing one place. Her Ego can neither individualize itself, nor reach autonomy. Anarchic persecutory experience and the presence of mortiferous persecutory archaic fantasies burden the clinical picture.

Jenny cannot constitute a straightforward neurosis because of the insufficient interiorization of objects. The emotional lack has granted access to an experience of isolation and dependency: a doubling of the imagos appears: *"All I know is that I do sports, after all this time I've spent with you, do you know who I am, because I don't?"*

CONCLUSION

The bodybuilder appears as the ultimate hero of the post-modern era. The achievement of athletic excellence and the condemnation of the continuous exploits that follow are often translated into the splitting and defensive arrangement of the addictive register. The culture of endurance to pain which permeate this society, potentiate the psychic vulnerabilities of bodybuilding candidates to finally reach the reign of the body. A muscle as penile substitute, a thorax for phallic succedanea, the bodybuilder brings onto his reified body identifications that compensate for his low self-image. To make his body visible, he kills it.

Synthesis: The interviews and analysis of the TAT of Sami and Jenny allow us to identify certain constants.

A negative evaluation of body image relative to a defective family, and a false perception of body image in comparison to a virile socio-cultural ideal of the physical plasticity, leads the adolescent to an exaggerated concern with bodily appearance. The subject is infatuated and he is plagued to a fixation and rumination. It is an act of dependency that is installed and is manifested through an adductive conduct: dietary restriction, excessive sports and dependence on anabolic steroids.

Synthesis 1. Adolescent body builder

–   Relation to the primary object insufficiently good
–   Object a-gaze lacking
–   Defective body image
–   Symbolic castration (maternal mediation and paternal presence) insufficiently accomplished; reorganized by means of another libidinalized and aggressive language
–   Unaccomplished identificatory processes
–   Probable homosexuality
–   Pathology of the narcissism
–   Passage to the act: dependence on sports and addiction to AS to hyperprotein foods
–   Body/ego ideal as reparation for the affected narcissism
–   Disorder of the imaginary register
–   Borderline of narcissism

Conclusion: A glorious body that fills the space with chest and biceps. It is an illusion of omnipotence. A permanent struggle against the voids of the gaze. The acquisition whatever the price of the Ego/body-ideal. Splitting of the *I* and the two bodies. Addiction. Bodybuildism is a pathology inscribed in the chasms of narcissism.

REFERENCES

[1]   Le Breton, D., (1990, 6°éd. 2005), *Anthropologie du corps et modernité.* Paris: PUF (coll. «Sociologied'aujourd'hui»).

[2]   Proia, S. (2007), *La face obscure de l'élitismesportif.* Toulouse: Presses Universitaires du Mirail.

[3]   Nasio, J.-D. (2007), *Mon corps et ses images.* Paris: Payot.

[4]   Lacan, J. (1966), «Le stade du miroir comme formateur de la fonction du JE, telle qu'elle nous est révélée dans l'expérience analytique», in *Écrits 1.* Paris: Seuil.

[5]   Dolto, F. (1981), *Au jeu du désir.* Paris: Seuil (« L'image Inconsciente du Corps se structure au sein de la relation désirante, langagière et affective avec autrui.»).

[6]   Nasio, J.-D. (2007), *Mon corps et ses images.* Paris: Payot.

[7]   Pope, H. G., Phillips K. A., and Olivarda R. (2000). *The Adonis complex: The secret crisis of male body obsession.* New York: The Free Press.

[8]   Winnicott, D.W. (1945), «Le développement affectif primaire», in *De la pédiatrie à la psychanalyse*, Paris: Gallimard, 1983, pp. 33 à 47.

[9]   Anzieu, D (1985, éd. Revue et augmentée1995), *Le Moi-peau*, Paris: Dunod.

[10] Lacan, J. (1955-56), «D'une question préliminaire à tout traitement possible de la psychose» *Ecrits 2,* Paris: Seuil, 1971.

[11] Green, A. (1979), «L'angoisseet le narcissisme», in *Revue Française de psychanalyse, 43,* pp. 53-60.

[12] Jeammet, P. (1980), Réalité externe et réalité interne, importance de leur articulation et de leur spécificité à l'adolescence.», *Revue française de psychanalyse, 44,* pp. 481-502.

[13] Assoun, P.-L. (2002), *Leçons de psychanalyse sur le masochisme.* Paris: Anthropos.

Chapter 2

THE MARKED SKIN

INTRODUCTION

" With ink I have written drawings on my skin. The drawings are of me. I came into the world without being anyone, and now I am Rebecca" (Poem of Rebecca, 19 years).

Psychic envelope, psychic skin, Ego-skin, containing object, containing and container, attracting object, terms so often used to say the skin.

A veritable organ to feel and think, the skin is a person's visible origin of identity, the incarnation of the flesh; one exists in one's own skin (well or poorly). Current fashion, tattooing the skin is an old story; an initiating ritual, a sacred and mysterious sign, an emblem of belonging and recognition, a racist seal. The tattoo, a corporeal mark drawn then introjected into the skin, presents itself at first glance: a drawing of recognition, an identification card. If in traditional societies these brands are a claim of descent, tribal, whether cosmic or spiritual, today the scarifications seem to have an individualizing function and, for some, even a social protest. However, beyond the current infatuation, seductive and eroticizing, as mentioned by Lacan [1], or the proclamation of individuality, tattooing may take on a more complex sense of a skin of replacement.

Starting with the containment function of the skin envelope, by anaclisis skin-Ego - an introjected figuration of the child's development from the experiences sensed on the surface - dedicated since Anzieu [2] and of what Bick calls the *second skin* [3] - constitutes a false self - we have conceived the idea that the marked skin, the skin-ego or that which wants to be the ego, is an intrusive and substitute skin.

In effect, the marking of the skin, a cartographic projective space of anguishes, or *tattooism* conceived as an instauration of an introjected and substitute skin-ego, already puts forth an interrogation about the child's search for another skin, his representations of containment, his integration capacities, his investment of objects and his emotional capacity for pleasure and pain; in summary, a questioning of his identity.

Through the lexical field of 11 adolescents (3 boys and 8 girls), illustrated by *tattooed* depictions, drawings that they choose and of which they speak, and two clinical case studies (administration of TAT and semi-directive interview), we analyze the *tattooism*, that is to say, the mark experienced as a distinctive sign, metaphorical object, representing the missing psychic envelope.

1. The New-Skin

"The instauration of the ego-skin meets the need for a narcissistic envelope and ensures to the psychical apparatus a certainty and a constancy of a basis of well-being [...]." [4: 39].

The marks and corporeal imprints, indelible, present themselves in various forms, drawing a thematic ensemble and appear on the skin of the back, shoulders, arms, legs, the lower waist, the wrists, nipples, sex, stomach, and everywhere else on the body, often accompanied by piercings. The decorated person who thinks of himself as the master of the work, decides the value of his body and, beyond that, the meaning of his life.

The semi-directive interviews with adolescents allowed us to identify the following lexicon.

The lexical fields of the adolescent *tattooists'* interviews first take hold of the body and its aesthetic sense. *"My tattoos have embellished me [...]"* (Nicole, 18 years old); *"I love my tattooed body"* (Joelle 17 years old). The aesthetic of the tattoo is often hidden, as if to keep it to one's self. A secret force emanates from it. *"My most expressive tattoos are under my clothes. [...]. They are signs that give me assurance. [...]. You can only see the one on my back, look..."* (Dimitri,19 years old). Hidden but also shown to those who ask, and exhibited to some, the *tattooist* shows pride in his tattoos. The incision thus takes on a function of significant tactile and visual inscription.

Table 2. Lexical fields related tattooism - identified from interviews

Skin and aesthetics		Theme	Mother	Father	Age of first tattoo
Arm	Tattoo	Needle	Abandonment	Control	Abed - 14 years
Body and	Form	Color	Absence	Distance	Amal - 14 years
Body	Beautiful	Drawing	Coldness	Impotence	Anna - 13 years
Ache	and	imprint	Deficiency	Weakness	Dimitri - 17 years
Back	beautiful-	Black	Disagreement	Violence	Gibert - 13 years
Shoulder	seen	Theme	Disenchantment		Joëlle - 14 years
Legs	Beautiful-	(serenity,	Hatred		Nicole - 16 years
Nudity	hidden	Phoenix,	Inattention		Rebecca - 12 years
Piercing	Decoration	rebirth, tree	Indifference		Salma - 14 years
Skin	Aesthetic	of life,	Insensitivity		Samar - 13 years
		lizard,	Narcissism		Sylvia - 14 years
		dragon,	Rejection		
		tranquility,	Selfishness		
		lacing, etc.)	Surveyor		
148		96	66	24	13/15 years

The visual function of the seductive notch is to ensure attention. However, when the stigma is hidden, paradoxically intrusive in itself, it acts as a screen to shield against external intrusion.

"The meaning of this tattoo is serenity; I really want to live it" (Amal, 17 years old). The corporeal mark has the meaning of an externalized spatial projection on the skin by compensation for the lack of internalization of the skin. The infant, so little reassured of his feeling of existence, cannot think, nor contain the emotions he feels. The body of his *good enough* mother hosts him, carries him, and transforms anguish and pain into bearable experiences. The baby makes himself understood through the body, and the mother responds to him through the body. Pleasant and unpleasant sensations, or the lack of sensation, may alternate leaving their binding sensory and emotional mnemonic traces that are more or less healthy and/or pathological. The pricking of the skin by indelible scarification, an introjected imprint, is there to remind the engrossed child within of the absence of the marking of the mother, the mirror of the narcissistic reflection: *"This tattoo is more beautiful than Mother"* (Joelle, 17 years old); *"When I'm angry, especially at mom, I'll stare at my tattoos in the mirror"* (Nicole, 18 years old).

Border and site of exchange, the skin enlivens. The first experiences of the skin have an identitary basis which, when defective, can lead to the formation of a *second skin*, a substitute for the first. *"I feel dressed with my tattoos. They cover me"* (Samar, 17years old); an introjected skin of pseudo-containment of compensation. *"If I die my body will be recognized among a thousand"* (Gilbert, 17 years old): the stamped dermis wanting to be recognized, authenticated, the relation to the marked body is then the link with the object of the externalized representation of the self.

This new-skin of replacement is not without pain. The incorporation of pain is researched, as an aesthetic value, as a label that acts by a compensatory mechanism, *"This one is the most beautiful, I have just done it* (tattoo on the upper left breast toward the armpit)*, it caused me the most pain. I do not usually feel much"* (Rebecca, 19 years old). Sometimes embellished with a piercing, painful pinching of the mark, reminding us of the auto-mutilating behavior observed in autistic children. An aggression on the skin is a determinant defeat of identitary disorders, "A real confusion of a subject unable to immediately determine the boundaries that distinguish, separate, and distance him, in fact, from his object" [6: 25].

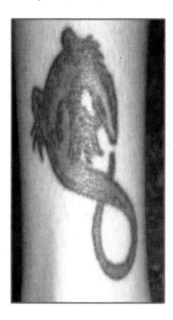

Figure 1. *Lizard* or *scaly skin*. A mythical tattoo of the legendary dragon on the ankle. The lizard holding its foot and tail to form a double circle (8 or infinity). The closure of the circle broken near the tail does not fail in reminding us of G. Haag's [5] circularity of the self - when in the failed acquisition of circularity, the child remains clinging to representative forms of rhythmic and turbulent oscillatory movements, like the lizard's tail (autistic movements). The mythical lizard, *"gives strength because of its scales* (skin)*, it seeks the light, because it comes from the sun"* (Amal, 17 years old).

The imprints tattooed are a fantasmatic representativeness of the object located on the skin space. The marked skin finds itself as such being the geography of the ego that is acquired by the experience of felt pain. Each drawing, each hieroglyph, represents a parcel, a piece of the ego; a part of anguish projected outward, fantasized and introjected into the interior, onto the self and within the self. The mark serves as a referent and a unitary substitute.

The notches of the epidermis correspond to narcissistic flaws. In all the interviews, there are parts of the tattooed body that are cited and with which the ego identifies, *"At first I had drawn the lizard on my ankle then I did the tree of life on my arm. I finally did the yin and yang, but what I like most is the phoenix on my back"* (Salma, 17 years old).

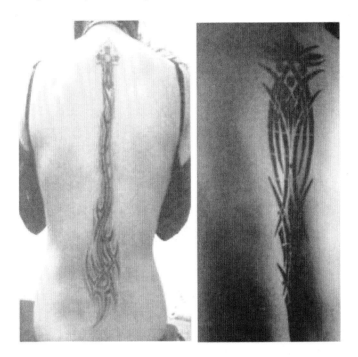

Figure 2. *Vertebral column* on the back. (Completely covered with tattoos on her chest, belly and legs, the vertebral column is the only one on the back of the young girl). This metaphor of the object refers us to the "the presence of the background of primary identification" proposed in 1981, by James Grotstein [9], which means the internalization of maternal arms that hold the back of the infant. Maintaining the back is a construction of the integration of its structure. The representativeness in this sense is an introjected auto-holding, *"Ever since I had my column, I feel that nobody can attack me from behind"* (Anna, 19 years old).

Bisexual identity, renaissance, differentiated corporeal narcissism; the imprint instills itself as a brand name, meaning and recognition. Each intrusive trace gives the subject a particular characteristic, certainly illusory, but which allows him to represent his skin to himself, *"I feel my tattoos"* (Anna, 19 years old*), "The tattoos give a meaning"* (Salma), *"I think without tattoos, one does not feel his body"* (Joelle, 17 years old), *"My tattoos are for me"* (Sylvia, 17 years). What, then, would not be hers?

Loss of the first object, rupture, abandonment, the mark is an epitaph, a sign of mourning the lack of the other and to the Other; but the imprints of that lacking other on the skin gives it an attribute of permanence.

"When my brother is sad, he looks at the sea to forget that he is angry, I look at my tattoos" (Salma); *"I feel that I possess something"* (Gilbert). Points of gripping and possessiveness, internalized identification, this clinging to fantasmatic representativeness is first of all a search for a fusional security.

Like the mother of the bodybuilder, that of the tattooist is non-containing: *"Mom has never held me against her"* (Rebecca); *"At school, when I was in kindergarten, it seems that I stayed for days and days before the image of a mother carrying her baby. I believe that even today I do not know how a mother holds her baby"* (Salma). Yet the mother of the bodybuilder is unstable, the one for whom the tattooist bears the image is the hateful mother. Klein said that hate is destructive [7]. It is on the model of this first object relation that the child's relationship with himself is developed, *"I do not like me"* (Gilbert); *"I think I sometimes hate myself."* (Salma); *"It is hatred of me"* (Rebecca).

Hatred of the mother is in fact deadly; she flays alive the narcissism of the child; based on the denial of otherness, the hate settles in the child the idea of self-extermination. The child de-subjectivizes. Maternal violence, hidden under the coldness, makes the child return this hatred against himself. Becoming the hateful mother by introjection, he tortures his skin as a separate object of himself, wounds it and then idealizes it through the denial of his aggressive act. He becomes jealous of the thing to which the mother gives interest. But this mother of hate is narcissistic and pays attention only to her beauty. The potentials of the child within closed horizons are returned against himself; an artist with impeded talents he notches, injures and marks himself. Violence and idealization are instituted upon the skin, the untouched skin by the mother's caress. The subject's field of power is limited to his skin area. But soon the tattooist becomes jealous of and competes with this idealized bedsore and repeats the wound for a more complex mark. And then, endlessly, re-begins.

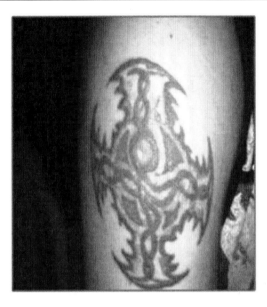

Figure 3 Tattoo of the *crucifixion* on the arm muscle, representing, in a circle, a crucified Christ surrounded by barbed wire (the framing of the circle). One can observe the injuries sustained during tattooing. The narcissism built from the psychical skin is tortured. This is not about the narcissism of the *divine child* [7], but that of the mortified child whose narcissism is essential for survival. This primitive anguish is annihilation anguish [8], an anguish of death. The metaphor of the object represents an attempt to take possession of the crucified narcissism through the intrusion of pain in the skin: *"It is the tattoo which most resembles me"* (Gilbert 18 years old).

This painful act exerted on the skin is linked to a primary ritualization that asserts itself as an organizer. Each point of the mark is a sensitive landmark, making us understand that the lacking skin cannot be approached, except through the intermediary of a rite. *"Every morning I run my fingers over my tattoos, to be able to go out"* (Rebecca, 19 years old) and to face the so frightening world and its absence of benchmarks. It is as if the obligated passage by the pain authorizes the access to the open.

Tattooists lack the space of speech, and the skin becomes that place, a space perpetually reinvented. The position of the good object is introjected into the skin, the *mise en scène* becomes imaginary, the symptom registered, the persecutory mother is soon indicated: the mark of the bad object is replaced. The mark becomes the telescoping of distress.

When hatred founds the relation, the arbitrary assumes power. The breach that opens is that of the fallen impulses. And all the subjects acknowledge that they have attempted suicide. Upon the maternal position defined by the splitter hate, the vital impulses are mortified and entangled. Will the father disentangle them?

The mother of the hate is unable to be the entryway leading the child to the port of the paternal metaphor. Symbolization fails and it is reabsorbed in the imaginary and transmitted to the skin. The father toward whom the child has stretched his arms is demystified. He cannot fill the gap left by the mother. Indeed, if the father of the tattooist is not the father of hate, like the mother, he remains the father of non-recognition: if his son recognizes him, he does not recognize his son.

If this doubling of the symbiotic skin makes its appearance during adolescence, it is because these epigraphs want to assert the difference, the ability to become independent of adult acquisition and to become an adult.

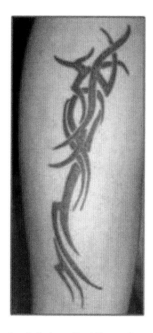

Figure 4. *Tribe.* Tattoo on the left leg. Braiding of non-existent links and lacking communication, the metaphor of the object is representative of the tribal belonging substituting for the dysfunctional family. The communication does not solicit the incapable child, therefore, to be the object and subject of links. The *alpha function* of the mother [10], the coherence of internalized objects, and the reference to the law of the father are deficient. The represented link becomes the representing link; the adolescent gives himself a fantasmatic linkage, *"I tried to get into a religious group, but surely my tribe gives me more security"* (Nicole, 18 years old).

It is as if the qualities of sustainability and identification are found in reference to another identifying paternity, *"These are my drawings [...] it is like my name"* (Abed, 17); *"My tattoos are here to tell my father that he does not control me"* (Gilbert, 18 years old). Signature of *I want to belong to myself*, by the use of the Name-of-the-tattoo - pseudo symbolic - as transgression of the father, the teenager does not want any other language.

"My father forbade us to play. We had to work with him in the field. I started at 10 years old. [...]. During the holidays, we spent 10 hours harvesting, and the worst part was the silence, since we could not speak. [...]. At 12, I wrote on a barrel, "The kingdom of misery." I think now it might have been my first tattoo," said Gilbert, 18, comparing himself to an empty and unaffected barrel.

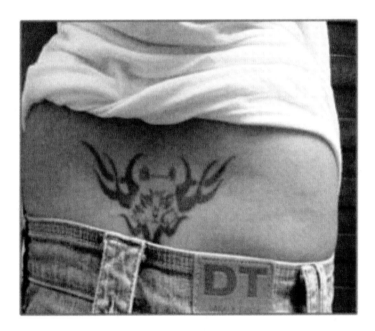

Figure 5. *The tribal totem cat.* The tattoo continues between the buttocks of the young woman. The complex representation is both tribal belonging and totemic protection of bisexuality, represented by the anality of the imprint. (Note that the cat is of two valences: a popular term to mean the female sex, it is here introjected in the lower back). This subjective position may also reveal, besides bisexuality, dysmorphophobic anguish in which the metaphorical object serves as protection. *"I prefer this tattoo to the others; it is my favorite and allows me to be tranquil and to be sure that my body is in good health"* (Sylvia, 18 years old).

"My father and mother were arguing all of the time. With my head against my knees, I wrapped myself in a cover so that I wouldn't hear them, and fell asleep" (Anna, 19 years old). First it is a cover and then tattoos. Both psychical envelopes of substitution for the young woman, the epigraph acts as a transitional object.

If the father of the culturist seems beautiful, but absent, the father of the tattooist is unsatisfying, his masculine identity is not strengthened, *"I do not know if it is the father whom I wanted to have. I would have preferred somebody stronger"* (Salma); *"I would have liked to have a man as father"* (Rebecca).

Identification processes therefore become laborious and painful, the passage to the Oedipus is difficult and bisexuality continues to play a role of the primary organizer. The subjective image of masculinity/feminity does not exclude a belief in psychic bisexuality. Through sketching, the adolescent wants to reclaim a body for herself.

The function of the spatial pseudo-envelope, of corporeal imprints, allows a projective and substitutive identification of what was not there. The necessity to build oneself an introjected skin while "the achievement of the symbolic barrier" is still unmet ensures the adolescent, through this "cutaneous prosthesis" [11], a restoration of the defective skin-ego, an ego-skin which, like the transitional object, is both me and not me.

Impoverished paternal and maternal imagos, family dysfunction, and the absence of recognition and communication weaken even more the psychical skin. Maternal containment and the paternal referent, the legend of the prick, possess form, theme and location that express the adolescent's illness of being.

The assembling of markings is an attempt at the spatial internalization of objects, involving maternal and paternal as much as the personal, a feeling of recognition of limits, a visualization of the body in its space in the world and a ritualized identity card. An illusory skin inscribing disorders of the imaginary register.

Lacking the primary egoic feeling, the *tattooist* clings to images to turn them into a history book and narrate his need to exist, to feel, to identify and to fight against his primary agonistic anguish. He makes a *new skin* to cover the gaps and burns of the psychic skin.

But his skin remains and he sees himself forced to the doubling of imagos: the skin he has, the clean skin that has not known the maternal fingers and remains untouched, that has not known the gaze of the father and remains unidentified, the bleeding skin from narcissistic chasm and the skin that is made through the wound of the stigma in order to hide the first, which he sees decorated in the mirror.

Shreds of the old skin always remain visible, however, which the tattooist increasingly makes disappear under new images. The Tattooism is inscribed in the pathology of narcissism.

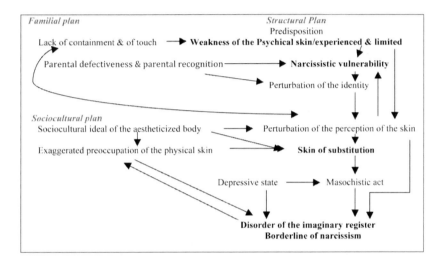

Graph 2. Schema of diverse psychological and socio-anthropological factors at work in the etiology of Tattooism.

2. ADOLESCENTS UNCOMFORTABLE IN THEIR SKIN

"The skin encloses the body, the limits of the self, it establishes the boundary between inside and outside in a lively, porous manner, as it is also open to the world, and vivid memory" [12: 13].

2.1. Rebecca

Rebecca, 19 years old, slender and of such small build that she looks like a little girl, is covered with tattoos (both shoulders, the lower back, the vertebral column, the right eyebrow, both legs on both sides, both arms, both wrists, the back of the left hand, the navel, under the left armpit, both breasts, the lower abdomen, the left ankle, the right buttock, the base of the neck, below the left-side of the waist) and with piercings (4 x 2 ears, the lower lip, the tongue, the navel, the left and right side of the pubis). Rebecca describes herself as an artist - she writes poems and *draws* her skin.

The father, an engineer who was working in Saudi Arabia, was not present at the birth of Rebecca that took place in Beirut. After the delivery, the mother, a Lebanese-Brazilian, had an epileptic seizure. Once she recovered, she returned to Saudi Arabia leaving the baby with her grandmother. The parents reclaimed the child three months later. A new pregnancy of the mother sent the girl, now 1 year and 2 months old, back to the grandmother.

The child grew up with her paternal grandmother who died when the girl was only 12 years of age. Three weeks later, the young girl attempted suicide, *"I thought that without my grandmother I could not live."* The following day, she had her first tattoo done on the *"left shoulder [...] this tattoo is my nickname, abandoned baby, but the others represent my renewal."*

Rebecca addresses the projective cards with attitudes of anguish and anger. The use of verbal precautions, rechewing, and hesitation between several interpretations in most of the TAT cards reveal doubts in the young woman, as well as her absence of certainty and assertion.

The projected perception that Rebecca has is that of a fragile and mortifying identity, *"An image that does not leave me is that of me as a child who is running in circles around my cadaver, being able neither to die, nor mourn."* The anguish of abandonment, of rejection, and of powerlessness, all of which are related to the oral phase, appear in the first card of TAT, through the story of a demystified then mystified child (c. 1: *It is a poor, lonely, starving boy, but he is a genius in music*). This ambivalence in terms of representation of the self could be a sign of a troubled identification process. It seems that, at the archaic stages, Rebecca suffered abandonment and precocious isolation. The obvious projection of the young girl on the card 13B (*It is me ... I always look for old houses in which to smoke and be alone*), goes back to a problematic of loneliness, and stresses on her avoidance and isolation, along with a certain confinement in the doing and the factual.

A remarkable restriction in the story and a spatial accuracy of vacuity, give to loneliness a dramatic meaning of non-integration of the superego, suggesting a possible split (c. 5: *Loneliness and empty house*).

The emotional expression of abandonment is doubled with phantomatization by her refusal to be seen or to have been seen and, beyond that, her refusal to see herself and to belong to herself (c. 16: *A child who is facing a mirror, but is invisible*).

Thus appears a doubling of the imagos: the maternal gaze reflecting to the child his beautiful image that was absent. This lack, that makes Rebecca search for her image in the mirror, is impossible to fill: the invisible always prevails over the visible, as she writes in one of her poems, *"I am the ghost who haunts your dreams."*

In addition, Rebecca's sexual identity is ambiguous. The castration of gender identity, *"If I was a boy my mom might have loved me"*, and fear of and for her sex, *"Both piercings* (around the pubis), *are the guardians of my sex."* Bisexuality appears in the story through a mechanism of avoidance and a confusion of characters: (c. 13MF: *a man wearing the clothes of a woman, she is naked and she closes his eyes so that he doesn't see her)* and in the following card (c. 3BM: *A boy or... a girl. ... In any case, he made a suicide attempt).* By the processes of negation, doubt, long intra-story silence and anonymity, the sexual ambiguity becomes depressive.

The compensatory search for pleasure through the corporeal imprints is clear in various forms evident throughout the interview, *"Only my tattoos give me pleasure."* The inability of the young woman to perceive and manage the boundaries between her inner and outer worlds (c. 19: *House? House and snow in the house, and two lighted windows in the black wall),* highlights her phobogenic anguishes and puts her in a schizoid position that the intrusive envelope, a transitional object, *such as the lighted windows in the darkness of the wall,"* still manages to limit. Indeed, she said these remarkable words during her interview: *"Without my tattoos, there would be no me."*

The family dysfunction is clearly apparent in the interview. The parental couple acts in an inadequate or even purely incoherent manner, *"I have never understood what my mother told me and I was punished for that."* Most times, the reaction of Rebecca is one of passivity, *"I used to hide and obey without understanding."*

Rebecca perceives her mother as a source of violence and fright, physical, moral and psychological punishments, *"she lashed me, insulted me and beat me."* This mother rejects her (c. 9GF: *A mother saw her daughter running away, but she turned her back). "My mother hates me,"* she says.

The relation to the maternal archaic imago of the splitting hate is a source of pathology. However, a maternal image of containment and care, *"my grandma, I loved her"* appears next to the frightening mother. In the good imago, there is a dominance of phallic objects in erection and bearing life, and in the bad imago these objects are in a state of stagnation and death. (c. 11: *A bad storm in the sea, a child drowned, but upstairs there is a door, it is not clear, and then there is a Phoenix...).* Rebecca's story is rich in altered elements within a perception of a bizarre detail (*phoenix*) reflecting the presence of one or more pregenital problematics. However, it appears that the image of the bad mother wins. The story (c.12GB) and the effects take us back to a bad mother/daughter relationship. The problematic of loss returns: (*There is no one in this boat. This indicates either that the people separated or that each one has lost their way or that they all died or fell into an abyss*). We can see an anguish of persecution that is related to the image of a devouring and castrating mother.

As for the father/daughter relationship, it is unsatisfactory, *"Dad didn't know how to be the father that I wanted."* Hesitation and regret appear in the story (c. 7GF: *A father sees his daughter smoking hashish. He does not do anything ... but what can he do? Nothing*). The father/daughter conflict does not appear, *"Dad was always absent. When he came to grandmother's house alone without mom, he was nicer."* The lacking father appears in the story through a direct projection (c. 10) that begins like this: *"A father and daughter, the father is busy.... She says is he going to come? She is also busy ... But this is not her father."* The Oedipal position is then recognized while it is avoided in the second card through the denial of links, but the denial and a double image, idealized and refused (c. 8BM), show processes that are completed with difficulty. The fabulated story outside of the image seems hesitant. The scotoma of the gun and the reaction formation, as a result of guilt, indicate the repression of aggression.

The parental couple appears in card 10, and is recognized as such (*a very old couple [...]*). The emphasis is placed on the relationship between the persons (*who remember the past [...]*). If the situation of the couple is manifest, however, doubt inserts itself and the threat of separation is underlying, *"one of them will leave or die, that is all."* Is she referring to her grandmother and her grandfather, whom she loved? It could be assumed, because she projects, in her saying, the imago of grandparents as *"an old happy couple,"* while her parents are, *"My parents, an odd couple."*

The analysis of the interview and that of TAT, strongly suggest the passivity of the father and the disinvestment of his function, and the maternal imago as a basis of violent and terrifying reactions. The family dynamics are organized around these reactions that render difficult the process of individuation and adaptation. Moreover, the doubling of parental imagos was the comparative support of two images, one good and the other bad, and refers us to the doubling of her imago. Often, a sexual ambiguity, or even homosexuality, appears making it difficult for a specific identity to take shape. The temporal precisions, by which we discover a problem of incapacity and

powerlessness, and spatial, which are centered around the unrecognized and avoided Oedipal conflict and around the ego-identity, are employed so that the subject can put herself at a distance of the character and the situation evoked by the cards, which arouse a sexual and identitary problematic that appears to be threatening: any desire whatsoever frightens Rebecca.

In the castration, strongly present and compensated by the valorized image of the decorated skin, an archaic superego, discernible through the representation of the bad castrating mother, prevails: *"I was always submissive and always froze in front of mom. I think I'm afraid, very afraid of her."* Thus it is also for the use of procedures in the story which demonstrate the restriction and avoidance of anguish found in all the cards related to the archaic mother: the long latency at the beginning of certain cards signaling the inhibition in relation to the maternal problematic; the splitting, (c. 2, 4, 6BM, 12BG, 13MF) reflecting in the equivocal good breast/bad breast related to archaic stages; the anguishing split affecting the ego, bringing Rebecca to the borders of the fissure of her identity.

Rebecca suffers from a dysfunctional family environment with an incapable father and an archaic maternal superego that are the source of persecution, abandonment and rejection, leading her to a narcissistic vulnerability. The maternal containment presiding over the psychic skin is lacking; it is only after a year and a few months that the child experienced a grandmother's tenderness. The frequent moves between Lebanon and Saudi Arabia, from one house to another, and from one mother to another, made her lose her benchmarks. The solitude in which Rebecca lived at first gives her a sense of isolation and powerlessness. These holes in the completeness lead her to a passive and painful corporeal acquisition: the *tattooism*.

The imprints of recognition that Rebecca injects into her skin are also revealing. The first mark was a message to her parents after the death of her grandmother: an *abandoned baby*, then comes the *vertebral column*, the back support that has not been recognized through holding (keen on tarot cards, she compares it with the blade of Death *"the column is also a head of wheat"*), and then in turn she marks herself with an eagle and a phoenix, representing the non-existent paternal protection, and then a tribal sign to give herself a family, followed by the epigraph of *"make love not war"* and a second tribal label and the pubic piercings, etc.. Imprint of recognition, epitaph, epigraph, label, protective signs, marks of belonging, and painful pricking, are all metaphors of replacement of the relationship to the lacking primary object; she is indeed *that child who goes round in circles*, and who does not manage to either live or die.

2.2. Gilbert

Gilbert is 18 years old, and he is the youngest of four brothers. The eldest has been diagnosed with schizophrenia, and Gilbert anguishes over the idea that he might also become schizophrenic. He is a timid young man at first glance, but once the ice was broken, he spoke slowly, always in short sentences, with caution and regular pauses. A first year university student in mathematics, he is always the first in class, he enjoys tennis, and he is passionate about jazz and keeps his headphones on all day long. He is convinced that *"problems come from parents."* He thinks he has *"problems with erection, out of fear."* His father, a man of the earth, was rigid and severe and did not allow them to play, *"We had to start working at the age of seven ... we were all in the fields, working, during holidays and vacations ... 10 hours of work daily."* He speaks of his mother as someone *"cold and mean, she has never kissed us."* Gilbert has around fifteen tattoos (1 x 2 arms, 2 x 2 shoulders, 4 on the back, 5 on the chest, 1 on the forearm; nothing on the legs).

The relations between father and son are sometimes tense, the father thinking that his son is ungrateful for the *"benefits"* that he lavishes on him, *"He thinks that I'm not grateful."* The son is angry towards his father whom he judges as *"very humiliating and hard on them."* He would have wished *"another father."* For the father *"playing and dreaming are a waste of time."* The children were isolated and did not see anyone, to the extent that *"a shepherd passing by was a joy to us."* If the father imposes the law of hardness, the mother seems a bad woman toward her children, *"We called her the witch, when we were little."* The elder of the brothers *"was forced to stay with her to work at home. [...]. He was like in a cage. Fortunately, despite the presence of dad and the very hard work in the land, we were in the fields."*

The projected self-perception that Gilbert has is essentially masochistic with a strong feeling of incapacity. A problematic of powerlessness is remarkable from the first card of TAT. In fact, Gilbert begins his story with an expression of depressed affect (c. 1: *A sad and anxious child who thinks about something. That's it*), and links his sadness to a mechanism of intellectualization with a general tendency towards restriction and the scotoma of a manifest object of phallic value.

Gilbert perceives himself as intelligent, but solitary *"I prefer to be alone."* The narcissistic defectiveness is strongly present. Gilbert seems inhibited, in need of help, but not daring to call out for it except through staring at the clinician. The affects expressed by the young man are mainly those of sadness, anguish, and unacknowledged anger. They are found in all the cards through a general tendency towards restriction, which reaches its maximum level of inhibition at the end of the test (c. 19: *Someone makes a drawing...*) through the use of framing and the brutal interruption of the story that has barely begun. These denote the fragility of the boundaries between the inside and the outside and his incapacity to contain his affects and differentiate them.

We find the narcissistic defectiveness combined with misrecognition of the self (c.16: *Each person is living a situation. We find people at ease and people not at ease. People who are thinking of the past, people are worried. I do not know*). Gilbert begins the story by putting emphasis on the actual; his thought here is confined to the factual and makes us doubt a dangerous evolution towards operational thought. The dominant affect is that of anguish. Thus, the adolescent refers himself to the external world and seems powerless in addressing his internal world. Gilbert projects the anguish of his vulnerable ego in an externalization process onto his skin. *"I do not care if Dad has a heart attack, my tattoos ... They speak of me. [...] I'd be naked without tattoos."*

Family dysfunction is clearly apparent in the interview. The evoked anguish is due to the non-expression of conflicts which weigh upon him as threat: *"I always wished to hear someone yell or protest, never. They're like the dead."* Nothing is linked and nothing is exchanged in this family, neither embraces nor emotions, words, nor cries. So it is, in card 3BM (*... an extremely depressed man*) that Gilbert, after a more or less long latency period, begins a very short story in which a strong depressive affect is recognized but it is not linked to an experience of abandonment or of solitude. The avoidance of the threat of abandonment and the tendency towards restriction allow us to assume that there is a problematic of inhibited loss. Once more, ambivalent affects stir Gilbert, leaving him in a state of lassitude. Fatigue has led him to the distress of suicide, *"But I'm not dead."* The family conflict, internal, non-said, has been crystallized on the elder brother *"he is schizophrenic because there is too much hatred at home. [...]. Both my parents are full of hate."*

The melancholic affects, not explicitly addressed, are linked to an anguish of separation. Thus, in the story (c. 6BM: *Two people waiting for someone, they seem to have lost hope, they expect something to happen, but I do not know what, that's all*), Gilbert begins with anonymity of the characters, and focuses on the anaclisis function of the object of negative valence; he himself seems hopeless waiting in vain for an impossible change. It is the same in his representation of abandonment (c. 13B: *Someone poor or a poor population or something old, he has poor clothes and is bare feet, someone poor, not happy with his life, we could say a vagabond child*). The problematic appears to be archaic and related to the loss of the object of love. What is the adolescent waiting for, what does he seek, what does he want? *"Nothing, only my studies and my tattoos."*

Poverty of maternal love pursues him and the imago seems to terrify him. The mother-son relationship is avoided in an archaic context and terrible doomsday: (c. 11: *I see hell! I do not know what it is, it is unimaginable! It is an atrocity! It is something that convulses and that is dying*). In this story, the depressive affect reveals a perturbed mother-son relationship based on morbidity and destruction. Morbidity, in fact, governs the relation; the young man evokes a bad object *(hell)*, and after an attempt of undoing he introduces an undetermined character who is not figured on the card, and uses an expression of terror. His is an infernal view provoking death, a perception of the archaic imago of the *hated* mother whose power is proven as mortifying.

The anguish of annihilation occupies the foreground of the subject's affect. In other words, the subject is unable to manage his affects and to have a satisfactory perception of the first object relation and then of his ego, which refers us to archaic movements that are destructive. Thus, at card 12BG *(the image of spring: something that is not old, I do not know what it is)*, Gilbert uses denegation with the impossibility to introduce an objectal dimension, which reveals an underlying narcissistic problematic of the ego subject. The archaic superego appears to be linked to control (c. 5: *A woman in her house, she inspects to see if she sees anyone in the room)*. Three verbs of visual perception invoke the image of the mother of hate, observer and examiner. A wicked surveyor!

The story of the adolescent is thus very limited at card 8BM (*It's something dead, I do not know something like that)*. Death returns another time, but the young man denies the morbidity of affect and avoids the aggressive aspect through the scotoma of manifest objects (*rifle and characters)*. He castrates the father, but does not tolerate the recognition of aggressiveness that is reflected on the self. In fact, destroying the father brings the child back to "the cage of the witch" in which is enclosed the schizophrenic brother. The hardness of the father is preferable to maternal hate, and the adolescent prefers to safeguard him in returning the aggression against himself - which reminds us of the crucifixion tattoo. The masochistic aspect of the drive turned against the self appears in the auto mutilation of the mark, *"I like to feel the pain of the tattoo when it is being done. That way I know that it belongs to me."*

However, the call to the clinician, the intra-narrative silence, the mechanisms of intellectualization and denegation, and the emergence of an altered projection reveal the presence of a father-son conflict (c. 7BM: *What does that mean? An elderly individual who is showing something to someone, he is explaining something to someone, I did not understand this picture well*). This antagonism to the father is confirmed by the anonymity of the characters and also by the intellectualization that holds the affective content remotely. In fact, the anguish arising from this relationship demonstrates a strong castration which, in turn, generates a repressed aggressive drive. *"I do not get along with dad no ... I must say I do not hear him."*

In the interview, through a reaction formation, a liability appears in the identification. The son refuses to identify with the father to the point of refusing his own identity, *"He is a zombie. That's why he could not bear his children alive. [...]. Surely they got the wrong baby at the hospital, I'm not his son."* Expressions related to an aggressive thematic of non-identification.

Although the father is harshly *"tyrannical and authoritarian,"* the Oedipal triangulation is not recognized and the conflict is avoided (c. 2: *A worker who works, a student, a housewife, a mountainous region. There are three cases in one region*). No link has united the characters who remain anonymous. The mechanism of isolation used and the numbered precision have the purpose of distancing the Oedipal conflict. Seeing the union of *tyrannical* father and mother *witch* is beyond the forces of the adolescent who governs by a manic defense: laughter, flip agitation on the card and again boisterous laughter.

This fright of the adolescent is found in the imago of the couple, as much in the interview as in the TAT. The interview lists avoidance mechanism, *"I have not lived with parents, but with a man and a woman, strangers."* The story is explicit: (c. 10: *Two characters presenting condolences, it seems they have been together for a longtime, or they are held together or brothers. Let's move to another one*).

The adolescent is struggling with the imago of the couple and begins with a representation of action associated with an emotional state of sadness (*condolence*) - death yet again! The couple is more or less recognized, but avoided (*brothers*), and so intolerable that the young man threw the card on the table. The parental couple, in fact, triggers strong mechanisms of avoidance and opposition (c. 13MF: *... This is a doctor visiting someone, I think ... this is all*). The adolescent avoids addressing the problematic related to sexuality and aggressiveness through the inversion of the drive and the scotoma of the naked woman.

In summary, the general tendency for restriction is raised in the story of all the cards throughout without exception: the long latency period, the intra-story silence and, particularly, the short narration. This inhibition on the part of the adolescent is particularly apparent in the evocation of father/son relationships, in that of sexuality, and finally in that of the imagos related to the couple. The anonymity of the characters, a procedure used in a large number of cards and specifically in the evocation of family relationships, gives us once again the perception of an adolescent who confines himself in his withdrawal, trying to avoid the projection of familiar imagos.

The representation of an object of negative valence (c. 4. 6BM) is a narcissistic detail that Gilbert employs to describe the maternal image. Raw expressions, affects of terror and morbid images describe the relation to the archaic object, revealing an anguish of annihilation.

Following that of the mother's, the paternal imago is anguishing and rejected: the framing (c. 12BG, 19), congealing the drive and impeding the access to intrapsychic conflict, the posture of significant affect (c.13MF) as a measure of protection against the emotional impact, the call to the clinician (c. 7BM, 10), the verbalization in the here and now of the administration when faced with the cards soliciting the *closeness* of father-son, show that the affect is recognized but is pushed back at the level of the external envelope. The adolescent refuses to internalize the identification to the father and externalizes the substitute for it. Gilbert, the tattooist, introjects his unwellness into his skin.

Gilbert has a difficulty in addressing his internal world, and manifests tendencies towards avoidance of conflicts. The adolescent confines himself to the factual, escapes in operational thought, and only manages to inscribe his ego in an imprint in his skin through a doubling of the imagos of his body. The narcissistic chasm apparent in his projections reveals the underlying existence of an affected representation of the self in its identitary foundations (Gilbert's prognosis is not very encouraging).

CONCLUSION

The maternal language of touch is lacking and replaced by one of hate. The paternal word of legitimization is defective and the adolescent resorts to an act of the body. The mark on the skin is a ritualized language of replacement, a painful touch and an overrated legitimacy that strives to be symbolic and hence remains fantasmatic.

A flaw in the recognition of the self through the alteration of the image of the skin and the search for recognition through an aestheticized socio-cultural ideal leads the adolescent to a depressive, even suicidal state. The subject obsesses, he is prey to rumination. The act of dependence is installed and manifests itself in a masochistic conduct: the tattooism.

The case studies of Rebecca and of Gilbert, the interviews with 11 adolescents, and their descriptions of the chosen signs reveal certain constants.

Synthesis 2. Adolescent Tattooist

- Feelings of non-belonging; search for a family meaning of replacement
- Feeling of non-recognition, search for an identificatory name of substitution
- Anguish of abandonment and frightening exterior, search for security and protection
- Archaic anguish, terror in front of the mother of hate; search for security and love
- Anguish of annihilation, search for sensation through pain and auto-mutilation
- Morbid feeling, search for references
- Relationship with the primary object lacking; search for an introjective containment
- Noncommunicability and isolation; search for the sign anterior to language
- Bisexuality
- Non-integrated law; search for limits and transgression through the signs
- Archaic superego, opposition and search for a ritual
- Affected narcissism; search for an egoic meaning through distinctive signs and use of markings as a transitional object
- Weak symbolic value; search for a metaphoric imago, and recourse to imaginary projections
- Defective psychic skin; search for prosthesis of replacement
- Disorder of the imaginary register
- Borderline of narcissism

Conclusion: An Introjected ink, an act of enjoyment which wants to be representative and represented but a metaphorical fantasy expressing the irreducible lack through doubling of the imagos. A suffering, an act of sensitive re-covering but substitution of emotional expressions; a new-skin, a skin for one's self created by the self, an ego skin, but a replacement for the identitary touch of containment; the marking of the skin is an attempt to identify, to introject the containment, to restitute a meaning; an attempt to restructure the narcissism.

The story in image of the *tattooist* begins with the primary abandonment and continues through the inconsistency of the referential; *"Loneliness and an empty house,"* as Rebecca says. The marked skin is an implementation of the ego that searches to be.

REFERENCES

[1]   Lacan, J. (1964), «Une des formes les plus antiques à incarner dans le corps cet organe irréel, c'est le tatouage, la scarification. […] elle a de façon évidente une fonction érotique, que tous ceux qui en ont approché la réalité ont perçue.» (p. 129), in Les *Quatres concepts fondamentaux de la psychanalyse*. Paris: le Seuil.

[2]   Anzieu, D. (1985 – éd. 1995), *Le Moi-peau*. Paris: Dunod.

[3]   Bick, E. (1967 – éd. 1998), «L'expérience de la peau dans les relations objectales précoces.» in *Les écrits de* Martha *Harris et Esther Bick*. Larmor: éd. Du Hublot, pp. 135-139.

[4]   Anzieu, D., Doron, J., et al., (2003), *Les enveloppes collectives*. Paris: Dunod.

[5]   Haag, G. (1992), «Imitation et identification chez les enfants autistes», *in* Hochmann, Ferrari et al., *Imitation, Identification chez l'enfant autiste*. Paris: Bayard, pp. 107-126.

[6]   Marty, P. (1958), *Les modifications du corps et de l'identité*. Paris: Payot.

[7]   Grunberger, B. (1971), *Le narcissisme. Essai de psychanalyse*. Paris: Payot (col. Petite Bibliothèque Payot).

[8]   Winnicott, D.-W. (1945), «Le développement affectif primaire», in *De la pédiatrie à la psychanalyse*. Paris: Gallimard, 1983, pp. 33 à 47.

[9]   Grotstein, J. (1981), *Do I dare disturb universe? A memorial to Wilfred R. Bion*, Beverly Hills, California: Caesura Press.

[10] Bion, W. (1962 - 1979), *Aux sources de l'expérience*. Paris: PUF

[11] Anzieu, D., (1985 – éd. 1995), op. cit.

[12] Le Breton, D. (1990, 5ᵉ ed. 2008), *Anthropologie du corps etmodernité*. Paris: PUF.

Chapter 3

THE MUMMIFIZED BODY

INTRODUCTION

"To make you become unrecognizable.
The remains of the donkey form a mask that is admirable.
Hide yourself well in this skin.
We will never believe, as it is appalling,
That it contains nothing of beauty" [1].

Enveloped in her donkey's skin, the princess escaped incest, and after pain and suffering, she has found love. The external envelope acts as a sterile field against the terrifying exterior.

The container is the place, the coherence for its contents, for their assembly, the space into which is linked the representativeness of the self (alpha function) [2]. This envelope is vital to development and if replaced artificially, can be favorable to the resumption of the evolution, at least in the lessening of suffering as *swaddling* cures and therapies using corporal mediation show us today. The enveloped body is remodeled and the sensoriality of this remodeling, giving meaning to the revival of the archaic containment, linking feeling and thought, sensation and the expressive speech. The envelopment can be seen as a final attempt to restore links. A symbolic space where the old lack and the archaic terror are faced again and assimilated.

However, our hypothesis is situated upstream. In effect, if *swaddling* cures may lead to a result, it is because they are supported by a therapeutic frame and word. If the term swaddling can introduce a regenerative dimension of containment, emotional release, *mummification*, swaddling the infant to excess already introduces us into morbid spaces. It seems that mummification, replacing the arms and the maternal word, is a world of silence in which the digestion of terror cannot be accomplished and links cannot be established; it can become a field of suffering, a space of self-smothering and psychical functions when used to the detriment of the ego.

Through the lexical field of six adolescents (2 boys and 4 girls) *mummified* at birth to excess for over a year, the linen envelope that is to provide security occults its goal and is no longer the metaphorical object representing the psychic envelope of attenuation of terrifying objects, but is the object of inhibition. We assist to a splitting of the body - the true body is the virtualized body and the perceived body is the one offered to sight.

1. A CONTAINER WITHOUT LINKS

"Movement is everything, it testifies to the psychical life, and it translates the whole of it, at least until the spoken word occurs. Before that, the child only has gesturing to make himself heard" [13].

Through mummification, the passage from the sensorial to mentalization occurs only imperfectly. The semi-structured interviews with *mummified* adolescents permit us to identify the following lexicon, through which we can see that the buried body language endangers the *alpha function*.

The lexical fields first take hold of the body and movement. *"Walking is beautiful, I go hiking every weekend [...]"* (Soula, 18 years old); *"They say I'm hyperactive"* (Nada 16 years old). The agitation and movement can give way to a state of asthenia: *"Sometimes I am tired, I hide myself, sometimes I'm in a state of great excitement, I have the shape [...]"* (Dania, 19 years old). But still there may be an attitude of harassment: *"I do not like noise or movement, I prefer to stay in my room [...], I stay with my Internet"* (Zyad, 15 years old); *"I spend all my time on the internet. I hate agitation and people and the street [...]"* (Candy, 17 years old).

We know, since Walloon, the importance of movement in the child's development. This development does not occur in a linear or continuous way, but we can schematically establish a progression. The infant's first movements are involuntary: around the age of two months he brings his fingers to his mouth, plays with his hands, smiles. He makes his first steps at 9 months and opens a door at 18 months. Around the age of two the child decenters and situates himself in relation to objects and to others, etc.

Table 3. Lexical fields related to mummifism - from the interviews

Body and movement	Nudity	Mother	Father	Period of the mummification
Body Body to me Freedom of movement Gesture Movement Skin Step Time	Collar Clothing Handle Hidden Nudity Seen Tight	Absence Coldness Deficiency Disinterest Distance Egoism Incomprehension Insensitivity Ignorance Narcissism Negligence Rejection	Absence Distance Incomprehension Laxity Unknown Violence	Candy - 1 year 7 months / day and night + 3 years / night Dania - 1 year 8 months / night and day + 2 years 6 months / night Hadi - 1 year / day and night + 3 years / night Nada - 1 year 11 months / day and night 4 years + / night Soula - 1 year 8 months / day and night + 3 years 6 months / night Zyad - 1 year 10 months / day and night + 3 years 6 months / night
104	67	31	11	

The first movements are exogenous, and then the child learns through movement, muscle tone, locomotion, gripping (autogenous) the ability to imitate and create movements leading to motor mastery and segmental movements. What movements could then make a child so completely tied up and what movements allowed him to apprehend himself?

The first function that movement takes on is the conquest of space from which the child felt himself cut off: *"I like to come and go and travel to new places"* (Nada); or that of her inhibition, a support of her phobia: *"It's silly, but I'm afraid of things that spin and roll. When I was little, I was afraid of balloons, boxes of matches, the pencil sharpener [...], I have never been to amusement parks [...] today I'm afraid of planes that pass, cars that go fast, the circus and especially of the big wheel [...]"* (Zyad).

The automatisation of movements is not gradual. The adjustment to the goal, the speed, and the rhythm are not necessarily mastered. Zyad suffers from stiffness in his gestures and walks in a jerky way. He is covered in bruises and ecchymosis as he clumsily *"enters"* into all the furniture. Nada has extreme agitation and cannot rest, she seems to dance without interruption, and she bumps into everything. Of the six adolescents only one, Hadi, seems to have a balanced approach. The coordination of movements (too much or too little) is questionable. Neither ease, nor harmony, nor freedom (Zyad) nor restraint (Candy) are apparent - Candy, paradoxically, knows how to draw, but not how to write, she wants to become a fashion designer, and she is ambidextrous-. If Zyad is afraid of movements that *"break him,"* he does not accept any imposed immobility. However, he is able to spend hours in front of his computer without moving, *"When the teacher said not to move, I wanted to jump on the desk. [...] I did not do it because I do not like moving"* (Zyad).

The infant, blocked in a swaddling cloth like in a shroud, the body wrapped, immobilized, isolated, enveloped by the silence, cannot contain the emotions it feels and cannot assimilate the terror of being. The mother's arms, which transform anguish into bearable experience, are replaced by a piece of cloth, *"When I have to wear a coat in winter, I feel depressed, it's like I am afraid of everything. I stay locked"* (Nada, 16 years old), who finds herself trapped in her anguish. The lively and warm skin of the mother is substituted with an inert mute skin, mute because the word of the link with the mother is also lacking. "[...] I recommend, especially for autistic children, making a sound envelope, which is ultimately primordial, along with the tactile envelope" [4: 36]. In the silence that is without maternal rhythm, thought does not replace emotion, does not link to its cause, and does not incorporate it. The world keeps an unspeakable and un-representable status.

The position of the absent mother/child link gives to the latter a posture of a passive receptacle. The movement is no longer what changes, what becomes. The temporal biorhythms are in turn distorted. The recomposition of duration is dramatic: what happened a year or ten years ago is confused, *"What time it is, I never know"*; *"I sit in front of my computer from the morning, and I only realize that it is night because I have to turn on the light, and I cannot see anything. [...] I also realize that I forgot to eat"* (Zyad, 15 years old); *"I have no notion of time [...], I only spot the moment when I have to sleep"* (Candy, 17 years old); *"I think I should live on a planet where there are neither hours, nor minutes [...]. A planet that is not round, but flat"* (Dania, 19 years old); a planet where one is not lost.

The false link of the envelope leads the child to a falseness of perception, which becomes observation and defense. The cloths have no eyes, and the mirror of the eyes is never there. A feeling of insecurity arises from the narcissistic chasm. The *mummifized* deploys permanent and exhausting efforts to feel what the other thinks of him, how the other misjudges him: *"When I go out, I get very tired because I'm always thinking about what others think of me"* (Hadi, 17 years old); *"If I see someone frowning their eyebrows, I think that it's directed at me and I try to disappear"* (Soula, 18 years old); *"I always feel that people are behind the scenes, and they see me while I do not see anyone"* (Dania, 19 years old). Fear of failure and rejection, feelings of persecution and avoidance, summarize the paradoxical fear of being seen and that of not being seen as well as the fear of being recognized and that of not being recognized. "If the mother's face is unresponsive, the mirror becomes something you can look at, but in which one do not have to look at oneself" [5: 203]. This hole in the image of the maternal gaze, the imposed immobility, the vigilant observation, and the wounded narcissistic integrity lead the *mummified* to an anguish of abandonment. To exist is to see to move, to feel; it is to make meaning of oneself through the other. However, for the child in the shroud, recognizing the world and being recognized are threatening, and the adolescent prefers "his planet".

In the absence of discovery through sensory movement, the structuring of reality and of the world is restricted, the schemas of causality, of permanence, of spatio-temporality are weakened, and the acquisition of representativeness fails; in summary, the substructures of future knowledge are delayed. The object exists only in the experience of the gaze, the only possible movement of the *mummified* child. What is visually perceived takes on meaning: *"I observe everything"* (Hadi, 17 years old); the imaginary built on the visual and the memorization that arises from it are considerable: *"I see an image, then another, a third, but sometimes I can not bring them together. [...] as an example, I see the door of the bathroom, then I see the shower running, I do not see the passage, I must make an effort to understand that I am going into the bathroom to take a shower"* (Candy, 17years old). The virtual construction is often a refuge for these children: *"The Internet is my world"* (Hadi). The virtual built becomes the transitional object, the toys, the alter ego, the mirror, the confidant, the communication, the book, and the knowledge of the adolescent. Because these children were unable to exercise motor skills in functional and fictional activities, they could simply build receptive games through their gazes.

This overinvestment in the virtual, a substitute for the gaze of the lacking mother, is doubled with a tactile overinvestment, a substitute for the skin, in the same way as oral overinvestment and under investment is a substitute for the lack of a nourishing breast, *"I am myself only at the pool"* (Dania, 19 years old); *"I spend hours in the shower"* (Nada, 17 years old). The waters of the womb are searched for and, when absent, the adolescent creates them: *"If I had to transform myself into an animal, I would be a fish"* (Hadi).

The problematic of orality is supported. Food is judged to be tasteless and is found to be underinvested, *"It is true that mom breastfed me, but she did so while chatting with her neighbors"* (Nada); *"I do not like to eat. I do it so as not to starve"* (Dania). Zyad forgets to eat, Soula is anorexic, Candy only eats soft foods, and Hadi has a bulimic purging crisis every Saturday. On the other hand, odors are searched for. They *"excite"* Candy who tries to find the origin of the aroma, and they are vital to Zyad, *"I cannot live without smelling odors."* However, Dalia has mixed feelings regarding fragrances: *"I am somebody that's a little bit weird, I love the smell of cakes, but I do not eat any, and I do not like perfume, but I wear some all the time."* Hearing is searched for and feared: *"I like certain noises, but I hate others"* (Nada, 16 years old); *"I seek silence, it is soothing"* (Zyad); *"During recess, the children made such a racket that I used to hide"* (Hadi). Maternal words, emotional expressions, and the story of oneself were not heard in the envelope of silence. The anguish of abandonment, in the mute and taciturn bag, gains ground, and what was supposed to be structuring is shattered.

An anal difficulty arises; these adolescents suffer from evacuation disorders; *"I was encopretic for a long time"* (Dania); *"I am always constipated"* (Zyad); *"I have learned to be clean at school because they wanted me out"* (Nada); *"I've been suffering from severe diarrhea since my childhood"* (Soula). Unexplained constipation and diarrhea are related to the excretion function and the feeling of incompleteness to which it is joined. The excrement, the body parts that are thrown away and disposable, prefigures the relationship to the mother [6]. The mother, assimilated to feces, may be retained or expelled. Bonfils [7] sees in it the development of an independent ego and the dual nature of the communication with the environment, with giving/retaining. In this regard, an essential feature of the object relationship is the feeling of losing a part of oneself: *"When I have diarrhea I feel that I keep nothing in my stomach,"* a void, a dispossession for Soula, the anorexic. A masochistic passivity of anal eroticism appears in these adolescents *"I was once taken to the hospital to get me to go, it had been a week since I had not gone to the toilet"* (Candy), as does a sadistic control of the object, *"Mom had to change me all the time because I dirtied myself, she told me that it was very tiring for her."* (Dania).

A narcissistic problematic appears for these adolescents in their links with the imperfect and fragmented object; the mother of the mummified is a mother of distancing and immobilism. The child is in the wardrobe envelope, but the envelope is not the mother and the mother is not enveloping; a lifeless container, with no words, no gestures, no eyes, and a living with no containment, no speech, no caress, no gaze. Unable to take full advantage of the object, a container doubled and split, the child finds himself in a narcissistic poverty which can put the integrative functions of the ego in check. The helping transitional object, "the narcissism allows the unitary completion of the lure through an introjective identification path - this narcissization will be even stronger than that which the invested object would have disappointed" [8:226]. The dead mother is unable to rescue her infant, and so the anguish is permanently installed. The mummifying envelope becomes a narcissistic shell, a transitional object, acting as a shield against the strangeness of the outside; but the ego remains caught in the compromise nets between itself and the object, and the object and the object.

With the objective of protecting their narcissism, the *mummifizeds* search for others, for love, for approval, for acceptance, and for affective dependency; thus quickly disappointed, they mourn for the object, and return to their shroud; and then start again. *"No one, no one answers me when I call, so I don't call again"* (Nada, 16 years old); *"I speak very little. I could die without calling for help"* (Zyad, 15 years old).

In these links, based on what is seen and without any further tactile support, the child feels guilty for the non-gaze from his parents, *"When I was little, I had a strange fear, I thought Mom was blind"* (Zyad); *" I do not want mom to see what I do because she will be angry"* (Soula, 18 years old). A feeling of guilt for the blindness of the mother does not go without reminding us of Jocasta and Oedipus. Could it be an incestuous desire that pushed the mother to cover up the admired body of the child? A possible hypothesis, according to the candid Candy sayings *"Mom is cold, but I think she is afraid to be kissed."*

The dead mother of the *mummifized* is, in fact, a *fetishist* putting between herself and the child's body a veil, fearing the desire. The fear of incest pushes her to install, between her and the child-penis, a distance, transforming the child into an inanimate object, reifying him. Henceforth fetish, the child can survive, and the condition to survival is to be a dead/alive.

The *mise en scène* of the *mummifized*, fetishized body is found in the clothing of the adolescents who are overly covered but dream of wearing too little, *"I'd love to live in a desert island so that I can walk around naked"* (Nada). The clothing has a social function: it is the limitation of bare skin in what it represents of the personal and the erotic, or a model (costume) of belonging to a group. But the clothing is a constant reminder to these adolescents of the hardness of swaddling, and then takes a particular meaning: *"I cannot stand wool, I do not wear it, it's too heavy and too closed"* (Candy). Or that through identification with the envelopment, they lock themselves into restricted clothing; Zyad, Hadi, Soula, and Dania only wear black and are always fully dressed in turtlenecks, long sleeves, skin-tight slim jeans and boots in summer as well as winter. Thus, their style of dress becomes a distinctive repetition of fetishization, and is stripped of adaptive functionality, keeping the limitation but without the containment: *"Clothes hide me. I feel like wearing an airy dress, but I cannot, I buy one sometimes, but I throw it away"* (Soula, 18 years old). The desire seems inaccessible, and although as *vaporous* as a dream of love, it is repelled, *thrown*.

The compulsion of clothes shopping is very strong, and the least amount of money is used to buy clothes. This form of addiction to clothing is an assurance of the invisibility of the body of reality as of the body of desire: *"I get dressed, then I am somebody else"* (Zyad); *"Why do I get dressed like this? Uh ... Because this way my body and I are hidden"* (Hadi); *"I always take care of my outfit, because with my clothes I can make believe I'm this or that person"* (Dania). Clothes are a staging dress, an optical illusion of the true ego; a cache-misery!

The hidden body is the fantasized body, invisible to others and only the adolescent knows it: *"This is how my body remains mine, nobody can touch it and spoil it"* (Soula); *"He who sees me does not know that he is mistaken"* (Dania). The distress of the fetishized by the mother is written in the distance: the body can be neither seen, nor touched, otherwise it would be *spoiled*.

Aiming to look like their idols, Emos or Goths, and to imitate their outfits, mummified adolescents cannot, inaddition, face the outside without a fetish bandage, often made of leather or cotton, on the body: on an arm, a leg, forehead, or on the penis.

In fact, it is not the clothing that is important; ultimately, it would not matter if it was not used as camouflage, or decoration, as opposed to what it really is. What carries meaning, and what the dress hides, is the velvet bracelet attached to the wrist of the adolescent. It cannot but remind us of the little bracelet of recognition which holds the baby's name and is put on the wrists of infants in maternities. This strip is actually a residue of their own fetishism, the relic of the virtualized body: *"I think that I show and I hide myself. My real body, I hide it"* (Dania). We witness a doubling of imagos: the *real* body is *hidden*, that is to say that it is lived as ghostly, virtual, it is imagined - only the adolescent can see it. The *shown* body, dressed is the meaningless body, a simple coat rack that others can see. The link between the two is established through this bracelet-residue at the wrist, a relic of the *true* body that allows the adolescent to recognize himself: *"I'll tell you, no it is not a leather bracelet, this is my ego, it is not for the others. This is what makes me smell odors for instance, or see people"* (Dania). Disincarnation of the body and virtual reincarnation of the ego in a ligature.

This relic of the maternal fetishization is overinvested in the function of a paternal substitute. Because the father, in this closed world of parallel persons, is no longer the father. His function as separator of mother/child, a function that presides over differentiation, has no reason to be here. He is an erased person, a simple echo of the divinity that imposes the distancing: *"For a long time, I did not know that I had a father"* (Nada); *"There was a man at the house it seems this is a dad"* (Hadi).

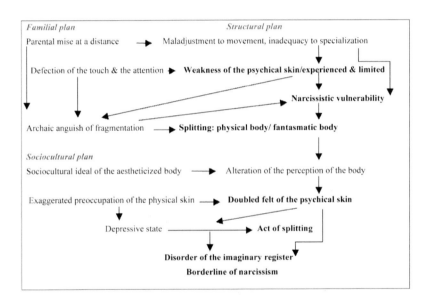

Graph 3. Schema of the various psychological and socio-anthropological factors at work in the etiology of Mummifism.

In summary, it is not the swaddling in itself that creates the anguish, but its representativeness. In other words, it is the fear of the fetishist mother, her fear of the desire, who isolates the child so that she does not touch him, that provokes the infant's terror and his incapacity to evacuate the dreads. Uncompromising mother seconded by a defective, suddenly violent father, who is wordless and submits to the sectarianism in which the child is engulfed. The movements of spatialization, of temporal rhythm, of the discovery of the real world, of the representativeness of the object, in brief, everything that makes up the life force is bullied, stopped, and fearful, the child is only half alive. He phantomatizes his body to safeguard it. Mummifism is inscribed among the disorders of the imaginary register.

2. TWO CHILDREN IN THEIR SHROUD

"There is no impossible mourning of an object in which the shadow is invested, but impossible mourning of an object never fully internalized and in which, consequently, one invests in the *hole* " [8: 161].

2.1. Nada

Nada, 16 years old, is the youngest of a family of four members. The father is an executive in a car sales company. The mother is the head of a bank department. She also has an older sister who is 19 years old and has begun secretarial studies. Nada is a junior high school student. It was only after 9 years of marriage that the first daughter was stillborn, then 2 years later the eldest sister was born, then Nada.

Although she does not ignore its purpose, Nada does the interview and the tests because she hopes *"to have a lover, and have the courage to talk to the boy who is courting her."* Nada's family is traditional and conservative, and the two adolescents are not allowed to go out. The only young people that they have the right to mingle with are their cousins. Nada thinks that she is *"a good girl,"* but she suffers from *"hyperactivity"* as she was told at school. However, she spends her days prostrated and locked in her room. The swing from one mood to another takes place abruptly and perplexes her surroundings.

Nada is dressed in ultra slim white micro fiber trousers, a sleeveless white cotton turtleneck, a wide black belt around the hips and high black leather boots. Twenty black bracelets are on her left wrist, topped with a white band encircling the upper arm; a wide band of black leather is wrapped around the other arm of the wrist to the axilla, four or five all-black collars are around the neck and five black rings are on the fingers. Finally, a lock of hair (Emo's Style) which enters the right eye complements her outfit. Having entered the consultation room, the adolescent does not take a seat immediately. She goes in all directions, sits, stands up, sits down, scrutinizes the clinician as if to gauge his intentions, sighs and begins to speak. Seeing me looking at her, she says: *"I'm prettier than this,"* words that seem trivial, but in Nada's comments take on the meaning of a splitting, in the sense that what I see is only the envelope that hides the body.

During the interview and the administration of the test, she appears agitated: leans back, folds over, crosses her legs again and again, fidgets with her ankle, triturates her fingers, fluffs her hair and shakes her necklaces and bracelets. Her vocabulary is poor, but her flow of speech is important and uninterrupted, the anxiety that appears beneath the comments keeps her on guard until the end.

Before every question, Nada starts talking. She talks about common places such as the difficulty that migrants have to live with - they search for food in the garbage, according to a TV show. A remarkable problematic of abandonment is noticeable early on in the interview and identifiable in almost all the cards of the TAT, related to the isolation and pre-oedipal stages: thus, in card 1 *"It is a sad boy, he is sitting alone, as if marginalized, he's looking at a paper on which there is something black."* The emergence of the depressive state in this card at the expense of the recognition of the anguish of castration, visible through a direct expression of affect associated with the emphasis on the sensory qualities (particularly a problematic of *black* to which we shall return), and through the final false perception of a strange detail without justification of the interpretation, as well as through the scotoma of the violin, shows an adolescent suffering from intense fear. *"I'm always worried,"* she said in the interview. *"Things can happen, like earthquakes, and everyone can die".* She links this fear to her mother: *"Mom was always afraid for us and that's why she forbids us from everything."*

The anguish of abandonment is dominated by inhibition: *"The kefulieh,* (linen for wrapping babies*), my mum enveloped me completely in it, it is mainly my arms close to my body that bothered me. It seems that the first two weeks I cried a lot, but eventually, later on, I became a good baby."* The banalized story of the card 6GF (*A woman sitting. A man who's smoking sees her. That's all*), ends with a veneer. The only link that exists between the anonymous characters, even in the structure of the sentence, is sensory *(see).* The parallelism between the two characters limits the relationship to an archaic voyeurism, to which was added a reference to oral dependency. This does not go without reminding us that Nada as an enveloped infant only communicated with the outside through her mouth that sucks and her eyes that see.

The gaze that forms the link comes back, repeated twice in the card 9GF (*A girl who is running, another one is looking at her. There is dirt on the floor. She runs fast, the other observes her*). The gaze at the object could have a paranoid significance supporting a voyeurism and a latent aggression, through a reference to anality, a problematic that appears for the second time after the black of card 1. Is not Nada the girl who is looking? Doesn't she feel like running, but cannot because she is a prisoner of her shroud? *"I would have liked to learn to climb trees, but Mom would not have accepted it."* The adolescent flutters, clenches her fingers on the card, crosses and uncrosses her legs, powerless to stop.

The anguish of abandonment emerges again in card13B (*A boy is sitting at the door, crying. He puts his hand over his mouth, he is sad*). The direct entrance into the story after a relatively short period of time reveals the abandonment, or the distancing, with an emphasis on the depressed affect, by a mechanism of rumination. The anguish is contained through the banalization and the anonymity of the characters. The anxiety to isolation is defined by a general tendency towards expulsion (*the child is found outside the house*), and by mutism (*hand over the mouth*). Nada feels rejected and unable to express her pain; just as the cries of the infant, calls of the magical thought which were supposed to have a power over the maternal presence, went silent, the adolescent cries no more, becoming with no cries, no tears: *"I don't know how to cry, I have no tears to let them flow. I thought at a time that it is an illness."* A false self is established, a mutism is installed. However, a reverse process takes place: the first week in kindergarten Nada did not speak, did not cry, and did not play with the other children. After the Christmas break, the teacher gave Nada's cap to another child to wear by mistake. The little girl snatched the cap from the child, threw it in the trash, and began to tremble and scream (the cap could be the residue of the packing). Since then, at school, Nada cried and was so agitated that she was given the label of *"hyperactive"*, a probable compensation for the infant's immobilism, but never again would she cry. However, although the adolescent chats sometimes today, *mutism* remains for her in the poor expression of affects and emotions.

In fact, communication does not exist in the family: *"Nobody listens to anybody."* The mutism seems to be a mechanism of avoidance, and it reappears in the TAT relayed by voyeurism; (c. 2: *A girl is carrying her books. A woman looks at her. There is a man who is growing herbs in the mountains. They are not talking to each other*). The tendency toward anonymity between the characters is intended to avoid evoking representations of oedipal relationships; the triangulation is not recognized in the absence of affective links; only silent observation unites the characters.

The white card seems to be a condenser of the adolescent's anguishes (c. 16: *It's empty*). The void of the white predominates internally. The avoidance process allows Nada not to express her anguish. The astonishment of the thought shows that she is going through an important emotional crisis.

The sensoriality problematic of the black reoccurs linked to a sexual representation. The shock in front of card 19 *(A house, snow, a tree, windows, a mountain in the side. A black cane that is coming down. People inside the house),* limit the story to evocation and rumination. We note the presence of short associations, of a false perception, and the juxtaposition of the limits. The description with an attachment to detail is a defense against the latent solicitations. The limits between *home/ego* and the environment (frame, distance, orientation) are juxtaposed, referring to a round-trip *(house/outside),* and indicating the failure of the trial for clarification. The *black cane,* personalized through a verb of motion, expresses phobogenic fantasies referring to a frightening penile imagery *(black)* and in motion, which prefigures a sexual act (an adolescent desire or a childhood abuse? We were unable to determine this).

The black of the cane is added to the black on the paper and the dirt on the floor: *"What's black, it's a lot of things, it is when we wear black because someone passed away ... that's when I hid in the closet, ... it's dirty things ... I do not know more,"* says Nada in the interview. Black is associated with morbidity, anality and with ignorance. The child in the dark and in the silence of his white shroud was powerless. Encopretic for a longtime, the little girl was at school *"ashamed"* of herself; but as we said above, the child exercises her power on her mother by the anal function and tries to evacuate her. In her anal fight against her mother, Nada sees herself unable to reject her because she is terrified by the absence of the relational, *"When I get diarrhea, I become empty... The emptiness scares me."* Similarly, the adolescent experiences herself as being incapable, the incapability even more anguishing because she did not know the cause: *"There are things I cannot do, can you tell me why?"* She said, in a call for help.

Maternal violence, verbal and humiliating, visual and terrifying, in default of containment and soothing words, was anguishing for the child who attempted to quell it, *"My mom reprimanded, she did not hit. Her eyes frightened us when we were little, it does not matter [...], I hid my face with my hands and my sister closed her eyes...."* is seen also in card 11 *(There is a sea, next to the stones. A corner. A crocodile),* the anguish is subject to avoidance in a banalized context with an enumeration in order to reduce tension. The non-evocation of the anguish is explained by a defense to the pregenital problems related to the mother, and the infiltration of thoughts through primary processes. The conflict refers to a superegoic breakage, apparent in card 5 (*The woman opens the door, she wants to check what is broken. She looks, and she finds nothing broken, there is a vase, a light, books, clothes well-hung... that's all).* Here also, the enumeration wants to have us believe that everything is reassuring, but in fact it expresses rumination; the adolescent opposes, to the searching and inquisitorial maternal superego, an attitude of denegation. The gaze again comes back with importance and takes on a persecutory value; the clothing, a false perception and the only term to which Nada has attached a qualifier conferring it a role as a good object, becomes a defense against the searching gaze. A fetishized defense allows her to hide her *real* ego.

The interview contains two assertions and three allusions to the mother's eyes: *"I dare not to say, mom gets angry, and if she gets angry, she looks at me and I have to hide underground,"* and seven allegations of neglect or abandonment: *"She forgot me several times at the door of the school,"* which clearly reveal the violence of the gaze of the mother and her tendency to put herself at a distance from the emotions and wellbeing of her daughter.

The relationship with the father is not less stressful by his absence and his inconsistency, but sometimes it is also physically violent. Nada only evokes her father twice in the interview, despite the insistence of the clinician, and mentions his nervousness and his violence: *"I never see him. I did not know he existed. [...]. He works a lot, that's why he is nervous ... and even more than nervous. ... He hurts with the belt."* The brutality of the father is present in the story of TAT; (c. 3BM: *A boy crying on a couch. His father hit him. He made a mistake).* The strong affect is linked to a representation of an abusive father, to a fear of loss (scotoma of the gun) and the recognition of guilt. The *mise en scène* of a persecutory character not figuring in the image, and the ambiguity of the wrongful (it is unclear who actually committed the *mistake*, the son who cries or the father who hits), the contiguity of the three sentences, and the lack of coordinating conjunctions between them cast the doubt - and Nada refuses to specify -, link the conflict and the depressive affect to physical punishment and promote the non-interiorization of the depressive position.

The emphasis placed on interpersonal relationships is inscribed in the framework of the relationship that Nada has with her parents. The adolescent suffers from a difficulty in adapting to the family situation. The analysis of the interview strongly suggests that the family dynamics are organized around the neglect of the mother and the mise at a distance she creates, and the violence of the father. The limits are inappropriate and the adolescent is in non-adherence. A negative emotional tone dominates, so does a mood of anger and hostility. Added details and misperceptions (c. 1, 9GF, 11) serve the dramatization. The representation of the action is linked to the state of fear and conflict with the object. The insistence on limits and boundaries is an attempt to delimit the space between the inside and the outside, indicating that the ego of the adolescent is fragile, even barren of its forces.

The anonymity of the characters (c. 2, 5, 6GF, 9GF) is inscribed in an effort to avoid the underlying anguish to the recognition of the protagonists of the conflict. It serves to camouflage Nada's guilt and aggression against the parents. In fact, it emphasizes the difficulty of identitary benchmarking of the young adolescent, who pushes the anonymity until the disappearance of the character and its commutation into a reified object (c.19).

The relation to the primary object is deficient. The adolescent is facing the mother in a defensive attitude, in particular in front of the powerful maternal gaze from which she tries to protect herself by the representativeness of the cloth (c. 5). The conflictuality with the mother is highlighted in a context revealing fear, aggressiveness and expulsion, through fixation to the anal stage; the importance of an anaclitic link is revealed in an ineffective attempt at marking the boundaries between the inside and the outside; there is an intrusion of the phallic object *(black cane)* into a contained inside. While the relationship with the father appears very negative, and the punishment to inflict on him outweighs the Desire.

The emergence of the primary processes shows that the persecution theme is predominant. Paranoia is manifested by the fantasy of persecution; the distortion of reality is found through the misconceptions and sensorial perceptions; the emphasis on the visual shows, on the one hand, the voyeurism of the adolescent, and on the other, an archaic sense of persecution; the massive projection is done through the perception of damaged objects, and the disorganization of thought through short associations. The only respite that Nada is given is when she is in front of her screen or with her music. Here, no persecution comes to disrupt her. The adolescent only takes pleasure in her fantasies: *"When I walk with my headphones on, I do not worry about people or anybody, and I travel to the stars."*

The identification is completed on a male centration (9GF) in a perfectionist movement. The anguish is more of a pregenital order, taking precedence over an anxious personality structure. Thus, the void of card 16 serves as a defense mechanism. Nada, who speaks without discontinuity, actually avoids verbalizing her fears and sufferings. The quasi-depressive attitude of the adolescent denies the possibility of expression; it is the astonishment of thought that dominates. Nada's ego is found threatened in its unity.

2.2. Zyad

Zyad is a 16 year-old, dark-haired boy, of small build, and, despite the fencing course he follows, he is rather poorly muscled. He is wearing black ultra slim pants, a black turtleneck with long sleeves covering half of the hands, large dark sunglasses which he buckled on his mid-length hair, black leather boots, a black ring on the right middle finger, a black leather bracelet around the left wrist that are relics of packing in which he was enveloped for a year and 10 months.

He looks clumsy and he is not always able to keep himself sitting or standing in one place. He changes from a state of extreme agitation to a settlement on himself, regretting that he is there, sinking more and more in his chair. He is silent, watching us through his half-closed eyelids, as if to gauge the situation, as if he is taming the scene, often throwing a furtive look, he makes three comments on the furniture, and asks twice if *anyone can hear the conversation.* It is only after a good ten minutes have passed that he agrees to talk, but in a laconic way and in short sentences.

Zyad is an only child, born by artificial insemination, *"I should have had a twin, but my mother lost it, and she stayed in bed until I was born."*

Zyad's father (44 years old), Bassam, who was the owner of a real estate agency at the beginning, is now only its director. The young man speaks of his father with a kind of animation, while his discourse is generally bleak: *"He does not always understand me."* Zyad finds his father moody and verbally violent, but only with him: *"He talks too loudly, he shouts, we do not know what to say ... but we end up agreeing with each other."* Physical violence is also present: *"My father is not a violent person, yet he hit me twice. I do not know why or when, once he slapped me, and another time before that he hit me with his slippers."* Bassam's violence does not seem to affect the adolescent who adds: *"I understand him."* Bassam's mother died in childbirth. Her sister (his aunt) took care of him. A year later, the father married her. Bassam has two half half-sisters he does not like, *"they are mannered,"* says Zyad.

Zyad's mother, Reem (39 years), is a pharmacist and owner of a pharmacy. She is successful in her career. The adolescent whispers, as if to avoid letting her hear what he is saying, and describes her as someone who is *"always busy. [...] She does not accept replies. [...] She does not like anyone to touch her stuff, or to change something's place. [...] She asks Mala (the housekeeper) for a report on everything, she wants to know everything in the smallest detail. [...] She is an observer, she knows it if we lie to her."* The son describes his mother as a *"neat, rather pretty and very, very thin"* woman. Cleanliness seems to be a major concern for Reem, and she is only concerned with her son when it comes to asking him if he is *"well washed."* Zyad is also *"excessively clean,"* and he is *"proud"* of it; moreover, he says, *"I was born by artificial insemination, it is cleaner as mom says."* This camouflaged allusion of the unconsidered sexual act gives us the impression of an aseptic child from birth. Unlike the father who shouts, Reem's anger is cold: *"When she scolds me, she speaks in a low voice, emphasizing each word, she scares me and I do not know what I have done."*

Moreover, Reem has never worn or caressed her son. She explained that she wrapped him in packing *"because it is cleaner."* Once again the notion of cleanliness is back again, and again she wants a rationalized explanatory cloth screen between mother and child. Tactile avoidance is repetitive in Reem's behavior and speech.

Zyad has a vague idea of the parental couple, *"I do not know if my parents get along or don't get along. [...]. I rarely see them together [...]. In the family we do not speak, we watch TV, and in fact everyone has one."*

Zyad thinks, *"that he is a little shy."* He has some friends that he knows from school, but *"I do not mingle with them a lot, because Mom does not like that."* At school, he is *"only good at history and geography, and very good at the computer."*

Zyad explains that his clothes are just there *"to say that I have the body you are looking at."* The (true) body for the adolescent is the one he has integrated in his fantasies, not the one we are looking at.

Zyad addressed the TAT with apprehension, becoming progressively more agitated with the cards. Visual sensoriality is substantial and the verb to see *(I see)* is used in all TAT cards in the affirmative or negative form, except for card 13B which elicits the question *"What is it?"* denoting vivid anxiety.

The analysis of the interview shows a family parallelism and relational modalities that are rather melancholic: *"My family is sad, we are sad, I do not know why."* Following the disinterest of the parents (except in respect to cleanliness), Zyad has no recourse *" I do not know whom to ask when I do not know what to do."* The overall emotional tone is marked by the dominance of negative emotions, sadness, anger and dissatisfaction: *"What's the point [...]. I feel like smashing everything. [...] Nothing can make me happy."* Zyad feels *"somewhat lonely and would like to cross the Atlantic."*

The isolation of the adolescent appears in the form of anxiety to the TAT. Thus, the direct entry into expression and the general tendency towards restriction in front of the card 13B (*A child is sad. Something happened. He lives in another house)* limit the story in a context of banalized depressive affects. The presence of two houses, one of which is suggested, leads us to a problematic of separation; however the anguish of abandonment is camouflaged through internalization *(live)* in order to avoid the loss of the object. In fact, it is a quest for an identity of the self and the lost object. The object relation is subject to caution, and the narcissistic wound is open. Zyad says it with poignant words and a feeling of strangeness: *"I wonder what I want to be and do. I get lost in my thoughts. [...], I do not look like the other boys much. I want to become a fashion designer."*

In addition, the boundaries between the inside and the outside are unclear or even absent, which also refers to a regression in the expression of phobogenic fantasies provoking inhibition of thought and preventing the development of the imagination; (c. 19: *What is it? What is it? I see a mouth and eyes. The mouth is big, it's ... it's a lion that is opening his mouth, perhaps to eat someone).*

The perception of rare and bizarre details and of objects that are not figured in the picture in which one is the bad object and the other is the victim, in an aggressive theme, reveals Zyad's anguish of being devoured. The test of the boundaries between the inside and the outside, and the good and bad breast, is questioned by a persecutory archaic experience with fantasies of devouring and cannibalism. Zyad is terrified by the terrible mother.

The shock at the blank page returns the story to an absence of structuration between the internal and external objects: (c.16: *What is it? Is it a white image? I see nothing! What is it, tell me? There is nothing!).* Zyad is unable to project himself into the white of the card. The interrogative affect-title reveals the emotional state of the adolescent in his quest to establish security and anaclitic links with the external object; it is not about a conflictual relationship between an inside and outside, but rather about a narcissistic defectiveness.

A double maternal imago appears in the young man that he tries in vain to reunite: the mother is at the same time the archaic object that he both fears and fears losing. Zyad speaks of an *"emptiness"* that he feels, and the joy he has to live his dreams, and quotes a poem by Verlaine that he retained by heart: *"I often have this strange and penetrating dream of a unknown woman who I love and who loves me, etc."* It is a dream of a tender and loving mother that is an unknown mother of his dreams by a compensatory mechanism. The anguish of annihilation and loss are highlighted in a banalised context in order to minimize the tension and the anguish triggered by card 11. Again, the object relation is wobbly, and Zyad is in an identitary quest of the self and the lost object: (c.11: *What is this? I see fallen stones and pebbles... Something, a building has collapsed. I see a woman coming down the stairs of the building running, ... people screaming ... Sometimes when the municipality does work in the streets, people scream).* The disorganization in the story, the instability of the boundaries between real and symbolic, the heterogeneity of functioning modes, the evocation of a theme inadequate to the stimulus, and the loss of logical causality are the signs of an archaic persecutory experience. Is it the ego of Zyad that is *collapsing*?

In fact, the adolescent experiences intense fear against his aggressive impulses toward the mother (c. 8BM: *Oh my God! I see a man, no it is a woman, she is watching two men in the shower, they want to kill a third who is tied up ... I do not know why. But it is the woman who comes in and cuts his throat).* This card, that revives his aggressive impulses of destructive valence, frightens Zyad who, strongly disturbed, attempts to protect himself by calling for divinity. The aggression of cutting the throat is a destructive fantasy emanating from archaic impulses: the lability in the identification, the bizarre spatial precision, the visual sensoriality, the raw expression with an aggressive theme, the denial of understanding, and the scotomization of the rifle express a morbid anguish related to the mother. Is he the tied up man, a baby tightly wrapped up in his blanket, who is killed? And does not he defend himself against death through the desire of killing its agent?

The fear of his own aggressive impulses appears in the interview in the form of remnants of the swaddling: *"I sleep under a mosquito net. I cannot sleep without it because, if I did, I'd spend the night killing mosquitoes, even if there is not."*

The adolescent also suffers from an anguish of castration, doubled with a feeling of powerlessness and loss of identity: *"I sometimes feel inconsistent."* Although perceived first in an artistic aspect, the phallic object of card 1 is related to a breaking (c. 1: *I see a boy, there is a guitar beside him ... is it a guitar? A violin? What is it? A broken guitar ... no, no, it's a rope that was severed. The boy in front of it, can no longer play).* The break focuses on an element, a partial object certainly, but certainly impeding the use of the whole object. The aggressive and intentional act of sectioning (by an assumed and unmentioned aggressor) has deteriorated the object, provoking a feeling of powerlessness in front of an act linking the ego and the object.

The mother, for Zyad, is a bad mediator. She unconsiders the father who, in her eyes, is *"a man who does not know how to impose himself."* Yet, Zyad is in certain *"complicity"* with his father when they go *"somewhere together."* But, why is there this complicity? Zyad says, with more vivacity, *"Daddy was here one day it was two weeks before I was 14 years. He looked at me and he told me: But your body, it becomes like a man now."* Should we see an eroticization of the father? Anyway Zyad clings to these words like a drowning man to a lost island in a sea of humiliations.

However, the rapprochement of father-son is a source of pleasure and conflict; (c. 7BM: *I see a man and then another, I see two men who are spying on and watching a third. They want to kidnap and kill him).* The conflict is avoided here by introducing a third party. The evoked aggressive themes introducing persecution, on the one hand, and the other, the visual sensoriality, alleging voyeurism, show a major conflict: the emotion relative to pleasure is linked to the anguish of morbid loss.

Zyad's conflict revolves around the recognition of his homosexuality. He is in search of it and is afraid of it (c. 10: *Zyad stares at the card, detaches his eyes from it, and stares at it again. What are they doing? I see a dead man and another one too, they are both dead, they go to paradise... in the sky. Someone killed them, but from above they know who killed them).* The couple is perceived in a homosexual register and in a mortifying context. Death allows one to be sinless and to reach heaven. However, would the intra-story silence and the repetition through replacement *(sky, for paradise)* allow for the assumption of another paradise, a sexual one, but undone? Thus, death becomes an escape from the image of the homosexual couple. Nevertheless, the evocation of a bad theme, the perception of a deteriorated object, and the religious reference make the desire of the father appear as a source of an intolerable conflict. Note the dead's capacity to know: the invisible perceives the visible that cannot perceive it, giving invisibility an advantage, prescience.

But this father can abandon him: *"When Dad travels, and he often does, I feel very lonely."* The anguish of abandonment related to the father generates sadness and depression.

The reversed Oedipal slope is remarkable in its link to a mortifying problematic (c. 6BM: *I see a man and a woman, they are dressed in black and they are sad, people pass by and offer their condolences. The father rather than the mother of one of the two is dead: they are offering me their condolences).* Gender differentiation is linked to an outfit of mourning and an affect of sadness. Zyad chews the same idea of condolences and through a slip of the tongue shows that he is the one who is concerned by the matricidal desire.

Notwithstanding the father's desire, Zyad uses defensive mechanisms of isolation against his homosexuality: (c. 2: *I see a woman holding books and observing horses. The woman looks well and sees, beside the horses, a young woman next to a man at whom she is looking. The woman is the mother of the young woman who is looking at the man, but there is no parental link with the man).* Zyad tries to place the story, which he starts on the manifest level in the banalisation, and makes a false perception (horses). The adolescent identifies the two female characters and isolates the masculine character. The projection of Zyad in the young woman reveals a homosexual position, which he wants to hide from his mother who *"sees everything."* Visual sensoriality is very strong, the mother surveys her daughter's look turned to the man, voyeurism finally denied and the adolescent does not want to recognize the link (parental) which unites the two characters.

While the sexual awakening of the adolescent is felt, it is however strongly inhibited: (c. 12BG: *I see a sailboat in a lake, a stopped sailboat and a tree whose leaves are falling on the boat, leaves and leaves and ... that's it).* The sexual act prefigured by the falling leaves, is suddenly stopped.

It is the same when it comes to the parental couple. Zyad gives a vague idea, by defense: *"My parents together! I do not think they have something in common."* The inhibition against the couple appears strong (c. 4: *I see a badly dressed man and a woman, and they are kissing each other ... and that's it)* and it persists despite the questions of the clinician. Neither ambivalence, nor the anguish of separation or abandonment are discussed in this story; the perception of the allied couple in an intimate situation is a source of enormous anguish that disrupts and inhibits Zyad so the adolescent attempts to intersperse between the couple a piece of clothing (man/clothing/woman) to which he gives a bad separation power.

The analysis of TAT and the interview provide information on the concept of Zyad's identity. In effect, an anguish of separation and the loss of the love object appear, as do traits of persecution and a weakening of the ego. We also find a confrontation with the external reality and the frightening object. The avoidance of reality and his confinement in the virtual *(and then I lose everything except my lap top),* and the refusal of intervention and the mechanisms of undoing and isolation express his struggle against depression and anxiety and narrates the maternal avoidance of the child's body buried in a linen. The problematic of aggressiveness against the maternal image, integrated into a conflictual story through an instinctual and defensive *mise en scène,* reflects the ambivalence of desire, stated in terms of life or death, as well as an identity disorder.

The conflict, as a mode of functioning, appears in generational situations and in the Oedipal conflict in the form of fusion/aggressiveness in the relationship with the parents. The inhibition is picked out; the anonymity of the characters and the restriction of responses (in most cards) show anguish and a defense against prohibited aggressive impulses. In all cards, an initial short-latency period and the direct entry into the story characterize the recourse to a dramatized aggression. The confusion of identities and the arbitrary search for the intentionality of the characters in the story are placed in a back and forth movement between instinctual expressions, defense, more precisely the avoidance, rumination and undoing.

Narcissistic defectiveness and anguish of castration predominate. Desire and sexual identity are both sources of concern. Here we find the fear linked to the relationship with the father as the source of desires and conflicts. Hence, the possibility of homosexuality.

Zyad gives the impression that he is adapted to the limits of the family frame, but seems easily attracted and fascinated by virtual models. This leads us to ask questions about the degree of containment (maternal security) and protection (paternal presence) provided to the child, and to formulate hypotheses about the precariousness of these links. Zyad says *"live by the spirit."* As long as he can build his world *"on the screen,"* that of his computer, but also that of his thought, he can *"survives all misfortunes."*

The anguish also appears in the banalization of responses, the hesitation in the answers, the chewing, and the interruption in the story due to the presence of an anxiogenic element. The perception of damaged objects reveals the underlying existence of a self representation infected in its identitary foundations, as well as the inadequacy of the theme to the stimulus, which is nothing but an escape of the manifest and latent solicitation for the benefit of another fantasmatic. The evocation of the bad object is, in the end, the projection that Zyad makes of his *"bad image,"* unbearable.

CONCLUSION

The sidelining, which prevents the development of movement, of the ensemble of sensoriality; a development of the gaze and the mouth, a false containment that mocks the real one: a blanket for a mother.

A delay and a flaw in the sensoriality and the conquest of space through movement and its symbolization, allied with an alteration of the body image and a double feeling lead the adolescent to a depressive state. The subject is prey to an anguish of *annihilation*, an act of dependence is installed which manifests itself in a conduct of rupture through fantasizing: the real body is split from the felt body.

Synthesis 3. Adolescent Mummifism

– Anguish of annihilation and frightful exterior; search for safety and protection
– Anguish of void; search for fantasmatic sensation
– Morbid feeling; search for benchmarks
– Relationship to the primary object lacking; search for containment
– Non communicability and isolation; search for the earlier sign of language
– Fear of contact but important voyeurism
– Archaic superego
– Affected narcissism
– Weak symbolic value; search for a metaphorical imago, and recourse to imaginary projections
– Doubling of the imagos of the body
– Disorder of the imaginary register; Virtualization
– Borderline of narcissism

Synthesis: The case studies of Nada and Zyad, and the interviews with the six adolescents, allow us to identify certain constants of a heavy picture.

This adolescent phantomatizes his body. What he shows is not for him but a parody. The body is split: one is fantasmatic, the true, the other is real, the false. It is the imbroglio of the imaginary, impossible to decrypt. Terrible suffering.

A hidden Skin, a defective image of the self, a *mise at a distance*, the mummifized looks at the course of things in life without being able to touch it. Fetishist splitter mother and expressionless father, the adolescent finds himself without symbolic or real protection. Virtuality becomes the story of his life. Mummifism is a new pathology of the narcissism.

REFERENCES

[1]   Perrault, Ch. (1694 – 1970), *Peau d'âne*. Paris: Classique Larousse.
[2]   Bion, W. (1962 -1979), Aux sources de l'espérience. Paris: PUF.
[3]   Wallon, H. (1941- 2002), Importance du mouvement dans le développement psychologique de l'enfant, in *L'évolution psychologique de l'enfant de l'enfant*. Paris: Armand Colin.

[4]   Haag, G. (2007), Les enveloppes corporo-psychiques, in Delion P. directeur *La pratique du packing avec les enfants autistes et psychotiques en pédopsychiatrie*. Paris: Erès, pp. 31-47.

[5]   Winnicott, D.-W. (1971 -1975), Le rôle du miroir de la mère et de la famille dans le développement de l'enfant, in *Jeu et réalité*. Paris: Gallimard.

[6]   Houser. M., (8ᵉéd. 2000), Les aspects génétiques – stades prégénitaux et complexe d'Œdipe, in Bergeret. J. directeur, *Psychologie pathologique théorique et clinique*. Paris: Masson, p. 5-49.

[7]   Bonfils, S. (1993), *Impertinence psychosomatique*, Montrouge: John Libbey eurotext.

[8]   *Impertinence psychosomatique*, Montrouge: John Libbey eurotext.

[9]   Green, A. (1993), La mèremorte, in Narcissisme de vie, narcissisme de mort. Paris: Les éditions de Minuit, pp. 222 -253.

[10] Freud, S., (1917 - 1994), Deuil et mélancolie, in *Métapsychologie*. Paris: Gallimard, pp. 145-171.

CONCLUSION

"I had no body, hence I made one" (Sami); "I had no links with anyone, I tattooed links, but what's formidable is that the tattoo has become my skin" (Rebecca); "To live I put my body around my wrist" (Dania).

Since the conception of the child, spontaneous motor activity appears to be synonymous with life and health. Some adolescents make of this statement a certainty in the mode of *I grow muscles, I tattoo myself therefore I exist*. The immobilism of the body is conjugated to the register of the unbearable. Others, forcibly immobilized, end up in the fantasmatic, the virtual, in the mode of *I virtualise my body, I preserve myself*.

The words of these adolescents, *"I suffer equals I feel; look at my skin do you know who I am, I hide and reveal myself when I desire it...,"* their recourse to a physical and psychical self-destruction, their feeling of distress, their affective, emotional and relational difficulties are revealers of their defective image of the self.

The shape of the muscular body of the bodybuilder, the pictured geography of the tattooist and the collections of rags and fantasies of mummifists can only express the vain search of the child who always wanted to compensate for the lack of love which gave him a poor image of himself, and to return to his body, his image. However, can the image he wants of a grandiose body, a populated body, a body of invincibility, really replace the image of a frail and unseen body, untouched?

The foremost relationship of these adolescents with their mothers is ambiguous, even persecutory. The narcissistic mother either imprints the relationship with her splitter instability or, hateful, she terrifies the child or also, fetishist, frightened of her own desire, she disappears in the distance.

Synthesis 4. Positions and imagos

Category	The non-containment		Imagos of the body		
	Mother Splitter Position	Father Anti Symbolic Position	Of the mother	Of the father	Of the Ego Narcissistic Position
Bodybuildism	*Instability*: narcissism and erotization	Humiliating castration Absence	Beautiful	Powerful	*Doubling*: Hidden body and muscled body, compensation and phallic substitute
Tattooism	*Hate*: Rejection and violences	Non recognition Non belonging	Beautiful	Inaccessible	*Doubling*: Dissimulated skin and marked skin substitute for recognition
Mummifism	*Fetishism*: fear of desire and distancing	Erotization Distancing	Non identified	Troubling (pervert)	*Doubling*: Dressed body and virtualized body, Defensive substitute to the fetishisation

The lacking gaze of the mother has printed in the infant a negative image of himself and his body, even for the mummified, it is an embryonic image. The huge anguish of annihilation incites the feeling of desertion and loneliness. Children become particularly vulnerable to the attitudes of the parents - detachment, neglect, rejection, hate, and fetishistic fright. The feeling of annihilation is rooted.

Linked to fundamental needs of security and recognition, this anguish is translated by a depressive state and an attitude of isolation and abandonment, and by anxious, aggressive or auto-mutilative behaviors. Against the abandonnic anguish, the child protects himself as he can. The feeling of powerlessness and insecurity generate violence or its opposite: the immobilism of the submission that can reach extreme dependence.

The relation to the primary object is thus confined within a context of inferiority, humiliation and culpability. The adolescent, not daring to face the culpability from his negative emotions, sometimes seeks to justify the persecuting, terrifying and castrating mother. Lacking mother, lacking body and unable to recuperate the first, he hounds himself in a masochistic position on the second. A narcissistic fragility hides under the glory of the visible body of the bodybuilder and on the skin of the tattooist. As for the mummified, he revels in the lost fantasy.

The relations that the adolescent attempts to build are doomed to failure. He tries to compensate for them by working on the modeling of the body; be seen and admired for being recognized and loved (bodybuilder), to give oneself a new skin defined and identified (tattooist), or to disappear, to virtualize (mummified) to protect oneself and survive. This new body is not the body of the self, but a realized body for the other in order to capture the admiring gaze, having failed to be the object of the loving and containing gaze. The body splits: there is the old body, the body of the reality of the self, invisible, hidden, under the muscles, tattoos or the virtual and the displayed body, exhibited for the sight of others.

The disturbance in the subjects' discourse and the emergence of disordered and altered projections reveal the presence of the conflict defective father-child. The father of the adolescent of the act is absent or resigned and violent when present, however, he does not permit a veritable access to the symbolic. Under no circumstances, he does represent a secure and protective authority: the law that allows the separation from the anxiogenic matrix and the law that establishes the limits of the ego. Under no circumstances, he does constitute a sense of recognition, a pole for identification, a social model. Under no circumstances, he does represent the healthy jouissance of the accepted desire defined in its limits. He is a man, castrated of his masculinity, a poor bearer of Oedipus: *"Dad is part of the human species, but he is not a dad"* (Rebecca). And this father, who is neither a Name nor recognition nor jouissance, engenders the vulnerable child with unfinished identificatory processes and an uncertain sexuality. The son and the daughter identify with the father's lack, with his undetermined sexuality. The sexuality of the adolescents is ambiguous and inhibited; their homosexuality and their bisexuality frighten them.

These adolescents have ex-corporated the bad object. The body emptied, bodybuilders have hidden their chasm with body sculpting, and have thus repressed threatening impulses, diverting them from their goal to make them harmless; the tattooists have introjected painful stigmas to give themselves a special recognition, an identity card. But the fetishized mummified can only virtualize his body and phantomatizes it.

It is no coincidence that our bodybuilders, tattooists and mummifized are adolescents. It is the juvenile crisis that has determined the choices. Their ideal of the Ego shaken by the lacks and rejections, both maternal and paternal, do not allow them to create a satisfactory image of themselves capable of supporting their wounded or deeply affected narcissism. Living this feeling *of disturbing strangeness*, they call for dependence and externalize their anguish in the search for the perfect, sculpted, stamped, or virtualized body. Therefore, narcissistic distresses appear returning them to the feeling of persecution, an archaic persecution linked to a hateful mother and a persecution relative to a defective father and to his weakness. The discharge of anguish is hindered, linked to object-dependence and the turmoil aroused by the changes in body image and the representations of the self. This paradox reveals the dependence on external objects, a probable reflection of the internalizations from childhood.

These adolescents are in a passive relationship with their bodies and to the fantasmatic life. The body becomes the representative of the objectal world, revealing the gaps of childhood. The threatened integrity of the ego, the hostility toward the object, humiliations and family demands, feelings of helplessness and disorder, the absence of recognition and non-limitation of borders, promote the corporal response which is made to ensure, through the exhibition, an access to self-assertion and a feeling of superiority.

The envy of muscle substituted for that of the phallus, the search for the mark substituted for the feeling of identity and belonging, the lust for the power of virtualization which has taken a preponderant place, are the witness of a narcissistic hole masked by putting in front elements of oedipal appearance. The screen memories revealed in their sayings, having conserved a quasi-persecutory force, attest in these adolescents to the existence of a split part in which the un-representable sexual difference is sealed. The acting seems to be a privileged means of externalization and protection.

The narcissistic corporal position that these adolescents adopt is in fact characterized by their defense in front of the fractured body image resulting from parental defectiveness engendering immature internal conflicts, and the absence of their gaze and their touch of the skin and the body. This fracture will lead them to develop, for the *mise in shelter* of the ego, strategies through a corporal act allowing for the (illusory) disqualification of the primary gaze of the parents upon the body.

Sport, the mark or the virtualization have the generating of emotions and desires for the other as their objective. The implementation of the narcissistic intention operates in a clear way in a seductive and virile mode in a denunciation of the non-recognition of the parent, and in a retracted way in returning the aggressive impulses against the self, through the instrumentalization of the bodies.

The disorders of sexual identity from which these adolescents suffer, weighed down by the massiveness of defense mechanisms, reveal that they have lost a part of their capacity to enjoy the feeling to be alive. Their anguish of annihilation would resemble that of autistic children (*"going on being"* of Winnicott). The threat from which they suffer is for not being able to develop the feeling of existence. In front of this sword of Damocles of the annihilating disintegration, they fight against the narcissistic chasm by the sensoriality of the action on the body.

The passage to the act of the body to the body therefore allows the avoidance of a confrontation with oneself, with one's desires and anguishes. It is then a search of corporal sensations by mechanical wheeling and dealing, muscular, programmed, or introjective aestheticized activities on the skin, but also imaginary movements of virtualization of the body. It is these sensations that replace the mental representations and the absent affects, and the imaginary that substitutes for the symbolic, granting to all these activities a lack of meaning foreshadowing the persecution and the corporeal narcissistic disorder.

In summary, the child lives between two parents who do not gaze at him, who do not see his body, who discredit him, who do not recognize him, who put him at a distance like a bad object, which basically is the same: denigration of the body of the child, of his being and of his meaning.

Identification with the aggressor the splitter, the child in turn does not grant any meaning to his body but uninhabits it; he disincarnates. Having become a bodybuilder he seeks to possess the marvelous body but despite his efforts remains outside of him.

The lover of muscles searches to transform his body into an enormous phallus that all eyes would be able to see. While the tattooist, wanting to reintegrate his body to possess it, to feel it, finally to recognize it, he forces it, hurts it and marks it. The adept of the imprint seeks to make his injury the brand name of his ego and exposes it to the eyes of others. The mummified, however, hides and virtualizes himself. The tangible body is only a clothes-carrier, whereas a relic of the mummification takes the place of the virtualized body. In order to achieve such performances, the adolescent splits his body and reifies it. The doubling of the imagos of the body is installed through mutilating the former body that has become invisible.

The search for surpassing the corporal limits of the body and its meaning, leads these adolescents to forget the organic reality to the point of rupture and pain. Their act of dependence appears to be the balm, the unique panacea for the narcissistic chasm *from when they were born.*

The person lives his own skins, he shields himself with muscles, with drawings, with tiny transitional residues and narrates, writes, scarifies himself; from surgery to implants, passing by the illustrated imprint or the muscle, he frisks his flesh, suffers, and so thinks of becoming a Man.

ACKNOWLEDGMENT

To you, who gave yourself a body and who has offered us these words, we dedicate this book of the body and these words of André Green:

"It is understandable that the object is both desirable and undesirable, lovable and hateful, and that the narcissist pole prefers to be than to have, though having strengthens the feeling of being" [1: 56].

REFERENCES

[1]   Green, A. (1979), L'angoisse et le narcissisme, in *Revue Française de psychanalyse*, No 452, pp. 51-5

BIBLIOGRAPHY

GENERAL WORKS

Classification Internationale des Maladies Mentales, (2002), CIM 10.
DSMIV (2002) APA.
Encyclopédie des sports, (2001), Paris: Hachette.

REFERENCE BOOKS AND JOURNALS

Abraham, K. (1917). «L'érotisme sadomasochiste» in *Œuvre complète,* volume I, Paris: Payot, 1965.

Akpo-Vache, C. (1996). *L'AOF et la seconde guerre mondiale : La vie politique (septembre 1939-octobre 1945),* Paris, Editions Karthala, (Collection: Hommes et Sociétés).

Altabe, M. N. & Thompson, J. K. (1995). Advances in the assessment of body image disturbance: Implications for treatment strategies. In: L. Vandecreek (Ed.), *Innovations in clinical practice* (pp. 89–110). Sarasota, FL: Professional, Resource Press.

Anzieu, D. (1974). *L'Epiderme psychique et la peau psychique,* Paris: Asygée, 1990, p. 266.

_____ (1985). *Le Moi-peau.* Paris : Dunod, 1995.

Anzieu, D., Doron, J. et al. (2003). *Les enveloppes collectives.* Paris: Dunod.

Assoun, P.-L. (2002). *Leçons de psychanalyse sur le masochisme.* Paris: Anthropos.

Beck, A.T., Ward, C. H., Mendelson, M., & Erbaugh, J. (1961). An inventory for measuring depression. *Archives of General Psychiatry, 4,* 561–571.

Bernard, M. (1988). «Esthétique et théâtralité du corps», in *Quel Corps? Corps symboliques,* mai 34-35, pp. 2-21.

Bick, E. (1967 – éd. 1998). «L'expérience de la peau dans les relations objectales précoces.» in *Les écrits de Martha Harris et Esther Bick.* Larmor : éd. Du Hublot, pp. 135-139.

Bion, W.-R. (1965). *Transformations,* Paris: PUF, 1982 (Coll. bibliothèque de psychanalyse).

_____ (1962). *Aux sources de l'expérience.* Paris: PUF, 1979.

Birouste, J. (2005). «Un regard d'addictologue chez les sportifs» in *Journal des Psychologues,* No 9.

_____ (1990). «Économie pulsionnelle du goût des sportifs», In: J. Bilard et M. Durand (dir.) *Sport et psychologie,* Paris: Éditions EPS, pp. 367-372.

Blouin, A.G. & Goldfried G.S. (1995). Body image and steroid use in male bodybuilders. *International Journal of Eating Disorders, 18*(2), 159–165.

Bonfils, S. (1993). *Impertinence psychosomatique,* Montrouge: John Libbey eurotext.

Bowlby, J. (1984). Attachment and loss, vol 1: Attachment. Basic Books, New York, 1969 & vol 2: Séparation: Anxiety and danger, Basic Books, New York, 1973; vol 3: Loss: Sadness and depression. Basic Books, New York, 1980.

Brazelton, T.B. (1983). *La naissance d'une famille ou comment se tissent les liens,* Paris, Stock Brelet-Foulard et Chabert, (2003) *Nouveau Manuel du TAT.* Paris: Privat.

Brodie, D.A., Slade P.D., & Riley V.J. (1991). Sex differences in body image perceptions. *Perceptual and Motor Skills, 72,* 73–74.

Brush, H. (1978). *The golden cage.* Cambridge, MA: Harvard University Press.

Burlingham, D. & Freud, A. (1949). *Enfants sans famille,* Paris, PUF.

Cash, T.F., & Brown T.A. (1987). Body image in anorexia nervosa and bulimia nervosa: A review of the literature. *Behavior Modification, 11,* 487–521.

Ciccone, A. (2011). *La psychanalyse à l'épreuve du bébé. Fondements de la position clinique.* Paris: Dunod (Coll. «Psychisme»).

Chiland, C. (1969). *L'entretien Clinique.* Paris: PUF, 6e éd. 1997.

Cohane, G.H., & Pope H.G., Jr. (2001). Body image in boys: A review of the literature. *International Journal of Eating Disorders, 29,* 373–379.

Collins, M.E. (1991). Body figure perceptions and preferences among preadolescent children. *International Journal of Eating Disorders, 10,* 199–208.

Corneau, G. (2003). *Père manquant, fils manqué,* Québec: Les éditions de l'Homme.

Davis, L.L. (1985). Perceived somatotype, body-cathexis, and attitudes toward clothing among college females. *Perceptual and Motor Skills, 61,* 1199–1205.

Dejour, Christophe. (1986). *Le corps entre biologie et psychologie.* Paris, Payot.

Decherf, G. (2003). *Souffrances dans la famille,* Paris: In Press (coll. Explorations psychanalytiques).

Dibiase, W. & Hjelle, L. (1968). Body-image stereotypes and body type preferences among male college students. *Perceptual and Motor Skills, 27,* 1143–1146.

Dolan, B.M., Birtchnell, S.A., & Lacey, J.H. (1987). Body image distortion in non-eating disordered women and men. *Journal of Psychosomatic Research, 31,* 513–520.

Dolto, Francoise. (1987). *L'image inconsciente du corps.* Paris, Seuil 1992.

_____ (1981). *Au jeu du désir.* Paris: Seuil.

Dutton, K.R. (1995). *The perfectible body: The Western ideal of male physical development.* New York: Continuum.

Emmanuelli, M. (2001). «La problématique œdipienne», in *Emmanuelli M. et Azouley, C., Les épreuves projectives à l'adolescence. Approche psychanalytique,* Paris: Dunod.

Fain, M. (1993). «Virilité et antihystérie», in *Quel Corps? Sciences humaines cliniques et pratiques corporelles,* pp. 56-64.

Fallon, A.E., & Rozin, P. (1985). Sex differences in perceptions of desirable body shape. *Journal of Abnormal Psychology, 94,* 102–105.

Festincer, L. (1954). A theory of social comparison processes. *Human Relations, 7,* 117–119.

Finklehor, D. (1979). *Sexually victimized children.* New York: Free Press.

Flugel, J.C. (1948). *The Psychoanalytic study of the family,* London, The Hogugh Press ed., Vol I.

Franklin, C. W. (1984). *The changing definition of masculinity.* New York: Plenum Press.

Freud, S. (1921). *La vie sexuelle,* Paris: PUF, 1967.

_____ (1916). *Introduction à la psychanalyse,* Paris: PUF, 1972.

_____ (1908). *Théories sexuelles infantiles,* Paris: PUF, 1978.

_____ (1905). *Trois essais sur la théorie de la sexualité*, Paris: PUF, 1967.

_____ (1917). *Métapsychologie*. Paris: Gallimard, 1994.

Gauthier, P. (1986). *Les nouvelles familles*, Montréal, Éd. A. St Martin.

Garner, D. M., and et al. (1983). Development and validation of a multi-dimensional eating disorder inventory for anorexia nervosa and bulimia. *International Journal of Eating Disorders, 2*, 15–34.

Goodman, A. «Addictions, definition and implication» in *British journal of addictions*, no. 85, 1990.

Granger, Luc. (1980). *La communication dans le couple*, Québec, ed. Sciences de l'Homme.

Green, A. (1979). «L'angoisse et le narcissisme», in *Revue Française de psychanalyse, 43*, pp. 53-60.

_____ (1980). «Réalité externe et réalité interne, importance de leur articulation et de leur spécificité à l'adolescence.», *Revue française de psychanalyse, 44*, pp. 481-502.

_____ (1993). Narcissisme de vie, narcissisme de mort, Paris: Les Éditions de Minuit.

Grotstein, J. (1981). *Do I dare disturb universe? A memorial to Wilfred R. Bion*, Beverly Hills, California: Caesura Press.

Gruber, A.J., Pope H.G. Jr., Borowiecki, J.J., & Cohane, G. (2000). The development of the Somatomorphic Matrix: A bi-axial instrument for measuring body image in men and women. In K. Norton, T. Olds, & J. Dollman (Eds.), *Kinanthropometry VI* (pp. 217–231). Adelaide, South Australia, Australia: International Society for the Advancement of Kinanthropometry.

Gruber, A.J., Pope, H.G. Jr., Lalonde, J.K., & Hudson, J.I. (2001). Why do young women diet? The roles of body fat, body perception, and body ideal. *Journal of Clinical Psychiatry, 62*, 609–611.

Grunberger, B. (1971). *Le narcissisme. Essai de psychanalyse*. Paris: Payot (col. Petite Bibliothèque Payot).

Gutton, P. (1996). *Adolescens*, Paris: PUF (coll. «Le fil rouge»).

Guy, R.F., Rankin, B.A., & Norvell, M.J. (1980). The relation of sex role stereotyping to body image. *The Journal of Psychology, 105*, 167–173.

Haupt, H. A., & Rovere, G. D. (1984). Anabolic steroids: A review of the literature. *American Journal of Sports Medicine, 12*, 469–484.

Haag, G. (2007). Les enveloppes corporo-psychiques, in Delion P. directeur *La pratique du swaddling avec les enfants autistes et psychotiques en pédopsychiatrie*. Paris: Erès, pp. 31-47.

_____ (1992). «Imitation et identification chez les enfants autistes», *in* Hochmann, Ferrari et al. *Imitation, Identification chez l'enfant autiste.* Paris: Bayard, pp. 107-126.

Haley, Jacy, 1990, «Changer les couples», in *Conversation avec Milton Erickson*, traduit de l'anglais par Brigitte CANIDESSUS, Paris: ed. ESF.

Henderson, L. & Wood, R. «Steroids: A fatal attraction» (2005). *British Society for Neuroendocrinology Journal* No. 1214, pp. 428-433.

Hertich, V. (1996). *Permanences et changements de l'Afrique rurale : dynamiques familiales chez les Bwa du Mali,* Paris, Les Études du Ceped, no. 14.

Herzog, D.B., Newman, K.L. & Warshaw, M. (1991). Body image dissatisfaction in homosexual and heterosexual males. *Journal of Nervous and Mental Disease, 179*, 356–359.

Horst, R. (1971). *Psychanalyse de la famille*, Paris, ed. Mercure Eberhardt de France.

Houser, M. (2000). Les aspects génétiques – stades prégénitaux et complexe d'Œdipe, in Bergeret. J. directeur, *Psychologie pathologique théorique et clinique*. Paris: Masson, p. 5-49.

Houzel, D. (1999). *Les enjeux de la parentalité*, Paris, ERES.

Jackson, A. S., & Pollock, M. L. (1978). Generalized equations for predicting body density of man. *British Journal of Nutrition, 40*, 497–504.

Jeammet, Ph. (2000). «Les conduits addictives: un pansement pour la psyché», in S. Le Poulichet, *Les addictions,* Paris: PUF, pp. 93-108.

Jeammet, Ph. et Corcos, M. (2001). Évolution des problématiques à l'adolescence. L'émergence de la dépendance et ses aménagement, Paris: Doin éditeurs.

Jeu, B. (1987). *Analyse du sport,* Paris: PUF.

Joiner, T.E., Schmidt, N.B. & Singh, D. (1994). Waist to-hip ratio and body dissatisfaction among college women and men: Moderating role of depressed symptoms and gender. *International Journal of Eating Disorders, 16*, 199–203.

Kaès, R. (1993). *Le groupe et le sujet du groupe.* Paris: Dunod.

Karger, Leit R.A., Pope H.G. Jr., & Gray, J.J. (2001). Cultural expectations of muscularity in men: The evolution of *Playgirl* centerfolds. *International Journal of Eating Disorders, 29*, 90–93.

Kernberg, O. (1997). *La personnalité narcissique*, Paris, Dunod.

Kimmel, M. (1996). *Manhood in America: A cultural history.* New York: The Free Press.

Klein, M. (1931). *Envie et gratitude et autres essais*, Paris: Point, Seuil, 1968.

_____ (1932). *Essais de psychanalyse 1921-1945,* Paris: Payot (Science de l'homme), 1998.

Kouri, E., Pope H.G. Jr., Katz, D.L. & Oliva, P. (1995). Fat free mass index in users and non-users of anabolicandrogenic steroids. *Clinical Journal of Sports Medicine, 5,* 223–228.

Kreitler, H. & Kreitler, S. (1970). Movement and aging: A psychological approach. In D. Brunner & E. Jokl (Eds.), *Physical activity and aging* (pp. 302–306). New York: The Free Press.

Lacan, J. (1964). *Les Quatre Concepts fondamentaux de la psychanalyse,* Texte établi par J.-A. Miller, Paris: Seuil, (coll. « Points »), 1973.

_____ (1949), (1966). «Le stade du miroir comme formateur de la fonction du JE, telle qu'elle nous est révélée dans l'expérience analytique», in *Écrits 1.* Paris: Seuil, (coll. «Points»), 1966, p. 111-180.

_____ (1955-56), «D'une question préliminaire à tout traitement possible de la psychose» *Ecrits 2,* Paris: Seuil, 1971, p. 565-600.

LaPlanche, J. (1999). *Entre séduction et inspiration,* Paris: PUF.

LaPlanche, J. et Pontalis, J.-B. (1967). *Vocabulaire de la psychanalyse,* Paris: PUF, (Coll. «Bibliothèque de Psychanalyse»), 1978.

Lebovici, S. «La relation objectal chez l'enfant», in *Psychiatrie de l'enfant, vol.1,* pp. 247-326.

Le Gall C., Martin, P. (1987). *Les familles monoparentales. Évolution et traitement social,* Paris: E.S.F.

Le Breton, D. (1990). *Anthropologie du corps et modernité.* Paris: PUF (coll. «Sociologie d'aujourd'hui»), 2005.

Lenders, J.W.M., Demarcher, P.N.M., & al. (1988). Deleterious effects of anabolic steroids on serum lipoproteins, blood pressure and liver function in amateur bodybuilders. *International Journal of Sports Medicine, 9,* 19–23.

Mac Dougall, J. (1989). *Théâtres du corps,* Paris: Gallimard.

Mahler, M.S., Pine, F. Bergman, A. (1980). *La naissance psychologique de l'être humain,* Paris, Payot.

Marty, P. (1958). *Les modifications du corps et de l'identité.* Paris: Payot.

McCreary, D.R., & Sasse, D.K. (2000). An exploration of the drive for muscularity in adolescent boys and girls. *Journal of American College Health, 48,* 297–304.

Meulders-Klein, M.T. et Théry I., (1993). *Les recompositions familiales aujourd'hui,* Paris, Nathan.

Minuchin, S. (1979). *Familles en thérapie,* Paris, Delage. Éric WILDMER, 1999, *Les Relations fraternelles des adolescents,* PUF.

Miollan, Cl. sous la direction de, (1995). *Parents et Adolescence,* Paris, Érès.

Mishkind, M.E., Rodin, J., Silberstein, L.R., & Striegel, "Biceps and body image", in *Journal of American College Health, 19,* 327–332.

Moore, R.H. (1986). «The embodiment of masculinity: Cultural, psychological and behavioral dimensions.», in *American Behavioral Scientist, 29,* 545–562.

Nasio, J.-D. (2007). *Mon corps et ses images.* Paris: Payot.

Olivardia, R. (2001). Why now? How male body image is closely tied to masculinity and changing gender roles. *Society for the Psychological Study of Men and Masculinity Bulletin, 6* (4), 11–12.

Olivardia, R. & Pope H.G. (1997). Eating disorders in men: Prevalence, recognition, and treatment. *Directions in Psychiatry, 17,* 41–51.

Olivardia, R., Pope H.G. & Hudson, J.I. (2000). Muscle dysmorphia in male weightlifters: A case-control study. *American Journal of Psychiatry, 157,* 1291–1296.

Olivenstein, C. (1983). *La drogue ou la vie,* Paris: Pierre Laffont.

_____ (1984). *Destin du toxicomane,* Paris: Fayard.

_____ (1987). *Le non-dit des émotions,* Paris: Odile Jacob.

_____ (1992). *L'homme parano,* Paris: Odile Jacob.

Pevous, et al. (1995). *Modification de l'image du corps et évolution de la dépendance psychique chez les toxicomanes.* Paris: PUF.

Pedinrilli, J-L., Rouan, G. et Bertagne, P. (1997). *Psychopathologie des addictions.* Paris: PUF.

Perrault, Ch. (1694 – 1970). Peau d'âne. Paris: Classique Larousse.

Petibois, C. (1998). *Dess responsables du sport face au dopage. Les cas du cyclisme, du rugby, de la natation et du surf,* Paris: L'Harmattan.

Pope, H.G. Jr. & Brower, K. J. (1999). Anabolicandrogenic steroid abuse. In B. J. Sadock & V. A. Sadock (Eds.), *Comprehensive textbook of psychiatry/VII* (pp. 1085–1096). Baltimore: Williams & Wilkins.

Pope, H.G. & et al. (1997). Muscle dysmorphia: An underrecognized form of body dysmorphic disorder. *Psychosomatics, 38,* 548–557.

Pope, H.G. & et al. (2000). Body image perception among men in three countries. *American Journal of Psychiatry, 157,* 1297–1301.

Pope, H. G. Jr. & Katz, D. L. (1988). Affective and psychotic symptoms associated with anabolic steroid use. *American Journal of Psychiatry, 145* (4), 487–490.

Pope, H.G. & et al (1994). Psychiatric and medical effects of anabolic-androgenic steroid use: A controlled study of 160 athletes. *Archives of General Psychiatry, 51*, 375–382.

Pope, H. G. & et al. (2001). The growing commercial value of the male body: A longitudinal survey of advertising in women's magazines. *Psychotherapy and Psychosomatics, 70*, 189–192.

Pope, H. G. & et al. (2000). *The Adonis complex: The secret crisis of male body obsession.* New York: The Free Press.

Porot, M. (1954). *L'Enfant et les relations familiales,* Paris: PUF, 8ème éd. 1979.

Proia, S. (2003). Destin du corps dans la cité: «Narcisse aux deux visages», in *Quasimodo*, 7, pp. 203-222.

_____ (2007). *La face obscure de l'élitisme sportif,* Toulouse: Presses Universitaires du Mirail.

Proia, S. et Martineau, J.-P. (2004). «Du surinvestissement sportif au gel de la métamorphose adolescente: Risques de décompensation dépressive et prévention», in *Neuropsychiatrie de l'enfance et de l'adolescence, 52*, 5, pp. 284-289.

Quivy et Campenhoudt, (1995). *La Technique de l'entretien,* Bruxelles: Université.

Racamier, P.-C. (1979). De psychanalyse en psychiatrie, Paris: Payot.

_____ (1992). *Le génie des origines - psychanalyse et psychoses*, Paris: Payot.

_____ (1995). *L'inceste et l'incestuel*, Paris: éd. du Collège.

Robert, A. et Bonillageut. (1997). *L'analyse de contenu*, Paris: PUF.

Rosolato, G. (1978). *La relation d'inconnu,* Paris: Gallimard.

_____ (1983). «La psychanalyse de l'idéaloducte», in *Nouvelle revue de psychanalyse, 27*, pp. 34-64.

Roussillon, R. (2001). *Le plaisir et la répétition. Théorie du processus psychique,* Paris: Dunod.

Seywert, F., (1990). *L'évaluation systémique de la famille*, Paris, PUF.

Shapiro, S. (1984). *A manhood a new definition*, N.Y.: Putnam's son publishers.

Smith, D.K. & et al. (1998). « Measurement of exercise dependence in body-builders » in *Journal Sports-Medical Physical Fitness*, No 9 (2).

Spitzer, B. & et al. (1999). Gender differences in population versus media body sizes: A comparison over four decades. *Sex Roles, 40*, 545–565.

Stevens, A. (1982). *Archetypes, a natural history of the self*, N.Y.: Pulitzer publishers.

Stern, D., (1981). *Mère et enfant. Les premières relations*, Bruxelles, Mardaga.

Terret, Thierry. (2007). *Histoire du sport*, PUF, (Collection Que sais-je ?).

Thompson, J.K. (1992). "Body image: Extent of disturbance, associated features, theoretical models, assessment methodologies, intervention strategies, and a proposal for a new DSM-IV diagnostic category—Body image disorder", in M. Hersen, R. M. Eisler, & P. M. Miller (Eds.), *Progress in behavior modification* (Vol.28, pp. 3–54). Sycamore, IL: Sycamore Press.

Thompson, J.K. & et al. (1992). Female and male ratings of upper torso: Actual, ideal, and stereotypical conceptions. *Journal of Social Behavior and Personality, 7*, 345–354.

Tomassini, M. (1992). «Désidentification primaire, angoisse de séparation et formation de la structure perverse», in *Revue française de psychanalyse, 56*, 5, pp. 1541-1614.

Valea, D. (2005). «Un regard d'addictologue chez les sportifs» in *Journal des Psychologues*, No 9.

Van Citsem, Ch., (1998). *La famille recomposée*, Paris, Érès.

Venisse, J.-L. (1991). Les nouvelles addictions, Paris: Masson.

Vigarello, G. (1991). «Pour une technologie culturelle dans le champ des pratiques sportives», in J. Ardoino et J.-M. Brohm (dir.), *Anthropologie du sport. Perspectives critiques,* Paris: co. Afirse – Quel Corps, pp. 146-151.

Wallon, H. (1941). *L'évolution psychologique de l'enfant de l'enfant*. Paris: Armand Colin, 2002.

Waser, A.-M. (1998). "De la règle du jeu au jeu de la règle: le dopage dans le sport de haut niveau», in Expertise collective dopage et pratique sportive, Paris: CNRS éd., pp. 20-39.

Williamson, D.A. & et al. (1998). «Eating disorders», in T.H. Ollendick & M. Hersen eds *Hanbook of child psychopathology,* New York: Plenium Press, pp. 291-305.

Winnicott, D.W., (1971). *L'enfant et la famille*, P.B. Payot, Paris.

_____ (1975). *Jeu et réalité*, Paris: Gallimard.

_____ (1960). *Processus de maturation chez l'enfant,* Paris: Payot, 1978.

_____ (1983). *De la pédiatrie à la psychanalyse*, Paris: Payot.

INDEX